# ESSENTIAL OILS
## AN ILLUSTRATED GUIDE

Mora iana.

# ESSENTIAL OILS
## AN ILLUSTRATED GUIDE

## JULIA LAWLESS

ELEMENT

Element
An Imprint of HarperCollins*Publishers*
77–85 Fulham Palace Road
Hammersmith, London W6 8JB

First published in Great Britain in 2001
by Element Books Limited

10 9 8 7 6 5 4 3 2 1

A catalogue record for this book
is available from the British Library

ISBN 0 00 712249 7

Printed and bound in Italy

## Picture credits

# Contents

# Preface

*Aromatic oils can be found in all the various parts of a plant, including the seeds, bark, root, leaves, flowers, wood, balsam, and resin. The wide range of aromatic materials obtained from natural sources and the art of their extraction and use has developed slowly over the course of time, but its origins reach back to the very heart of the earliest civilizations. The last two decades have seen a growing interest in complementary healing methods and the use of naturally derived products such as essential oils. Aromatherapy, once considered a fringe practice, has become so generally accepted and respected that it is increasingly on offer to hospital patients as part of their treatment. More and more, manufacturers of health products, cosmetics, and perfumes are recognizing the value of essential oils in enhancing the quality and appeal of their products. At the same time, the home use of essential oils has risen dramatically as people discover for themselves the therapeutic benefits and unique esthetic enjoyment of the oils. Current scientific research into the chemistry and medicinal use of certain essential oils has helped confirm and clarify their precise healing potential. The demand for tea tree oil, for example, has expanded enormously over the last few years as a result of detailed analytical trials – in Australia it has even been hailed as the "antiseptic of the future"! Such studies have highlighted the benefits of essential oils and the need for further research. Cultivation methods, climate, location, precise botanical species, extraction techniques, and handling have all been found to have a profound influence on the final makeup of an oil, thus affecting its fragrance, purity, and therapeutic value.*

ABOVE *The leaf of the grapefruit tree. Grapefruit oil is a valuable protection against infection.*

ABOVE *Sweet almond oil is made by pressing almond kernels.*

BELOW *Oil from mandarin leaves is used to strengthen digestive functions.*

# How to Use This Book

*Essential Oils* provides a general introduction to aromatics, showing their changing role throughout history and their modern applications in aromatherapy, herbalism, and perfumery. A therapeutic index lists common complaints, which are grouped according to different parts of the body, with information on how they can be treated using aromatherapy oils. A systematic survey of over 160 essential oils, shown in alphabetical order according to the Latin names of the plants from which they are derived, provides a comprehensive guide, detailing extraction methods, chemistry, and pharmacology.

BELOW *As well as discussing the origins and history of aromatherapy, the first part of the book shows you how to use essential oils at home.*

*Information boxes explain how essential oils work in different parts of the body*

BELOW *The Therapeutic Index groups ailments according to body systems and lists recommended oils to provide a comprehensive guide to treatment.*

*Abbreviations indicate the suggested method of application. For key, see page 28*

*Comprehensive lists of essential oils, grouped by ailment, are an easy-to-follow guide to home use*

RIGHT *The last part of the book lists 160 essential oils. It indicates how each oil can be used at home, how it was extracted, and with what other oils it is compatible.*

*This section details the various complaints, listed by body system, that the oil can treat*

*Special attention should be paid to the Safety Data on each oil*

# Historical Roots

AROMATIC PLANTS AND OILS *have been used for thousands of years, as incense, perfumes, and cosmetics, and for medical and culinary applications. Natural aromatics and perfume materials were among the earliest trade items of the ancient world, being rare and highly prized. When the Jewish people began their exodus from Egypt to Israel around 1240* BCE, *they took many gums and oils with them, together with knowledge of their use. In most early cultures the religious and therapeutic roles of aromatic oils were intertwined. This type of practice is still in evidence: in the East, purifying sprigs of juniper are burned in Tibetan temples; in the West, frankincense is used during the Roman Catholic mass.*

## ANCIENT CIVILIZATIONS

The Vedic literature of India, dating from around 2000 BCE, lists over 700 substances including cinnamon, spikenard, ginger, myrrh, cilantro, and sandalwood. But aromatics were considered to be more than just perfumes, and the *Rig Veda* codified their use for both liturgical and therapeutic purposes. The traditional Indian or Ayurvedic system of medicine developed from this understanding of plant lore.

The Chinese also have an ancient herbal tradition that accompanies the practice of acupuncture, the earliest records being in the *Yellow Emperor's Book of Internal Medicine* dating from around 2000 BCE.

But perhaps the most famous and richest associations with the first aromatic materials are found in ancient Egypt. The use of many medicinal herbs is recorded in papyrus manuscripts from the reign of Khufu, around 2800 BCE. Aromatic gums and oils such as cedar and myrrh were used in the embalming process, and the Egyptians were famous for their herbal preparations and ointments.

## TREASURES FROM THE EAST

Phoenician merchants brought camphor from China, cinnamon from India, gums from Arabia, and rose from Syria to the civilizations of Greece and Rome. The Greeks learned about perfumery and natural therapeutics from the Egyptians. Herodotus recorded the method of distillation of turpentine in about 425 BCE. Hippocrates, born in Greece in about 460 BCE and revered as the father of medicine, prescribed perfumed fumigations and fomentations.

The Romans were lavish in their use of perfumes, which they used on their hair, bodies, clothes, and beds, and for massage. Roman knowledge of oils spread to Constantinople, where great works were translated into Persian and Arabic and passed on through the Arab world.

LEFT *In the East, aromatics and perfumes were highly valued commodities used in sacred rites and offered in homage to the gods. This painting by Albrecht Dürer shows the Magi bringing gifts of frankincense and myrrh to the baby Jesus.*

## ALCHEMY

The "perfumes of Arabia" spread to Europe at the time of the crusades and became famous throughout Europe. Gradually, the Europeans began to experiment with their own native herbs, such as lavender, sage, and rosemary, which were used for strewing floors and as protection against plague and other infections. Distillation, used to produce pure essential oils and aromatic water, was employed in the practice of alchemy, the hermetic pursuit dedicated to the transformation of base metals into gold, a religious quest in which the stages of distillation were equated with stages of an inner psychic transmutation.

ABOVE *This eighteenth-century painting by Joseph Wright portrays the alchemist's equipment. Retorts and stills were used to extract volatile oils. The stages of distillation were equated with the purified human psyche by alchemists.*

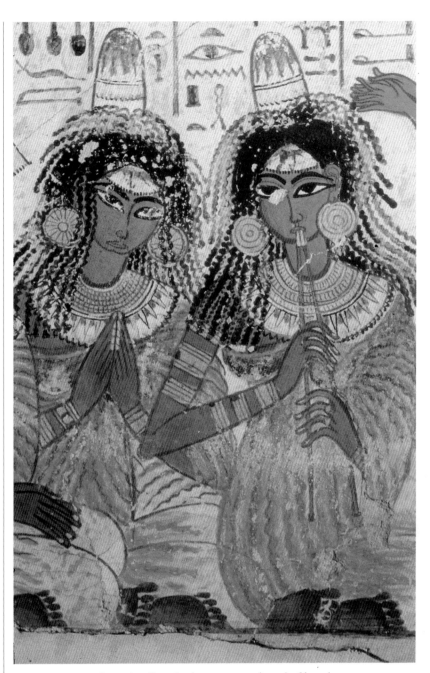

ABOVE *An ancient Egyptian banquet scene, from the fifteenth century BCE, shows women wearing perfume cones on their heads. As the heat melted the cones, their hair and bodies would be waxed and scented.*

## THE SCIENTIFIC REVOLUTION

For many centuries, aromatic materials were the main protection against epidemics. The medicinal properties and applications of increasing numbers of new essential oils were analyzed and recorded by the pharmacists. With the scientific revolution of the early nineteenth century, chemists were able to identify the various constituents of the oils and give them specific names. This laid the groundwork for the development of the oils' synthetic counterparts and the growth of the modern drug industry. By the mid twentieth century, essential oils were used only in perfumes, cosmetics, and foodstuffs.

# The Birth of Aromatherapy

THE TERM "AROMATHERAPY" *was first coined in 1928 by René-Maurice Gattefossé, a French chemist working in his family's perfumery business. He became fascinated with the therapeutic possibilities of the oils after discovering by accident that lavender was able to heal a severe burn on his hand quite rapidly and help prevent scarring. He also confirmed the discoveries made by Cuthbert Hall in 1904, that many of the essential oils were more effective in their totality than their synthetic substitutes or their isolated active ingredients.*

## HERBAL MEDICINE

Aromatherapy is part of the larger field of herbal medicine. The essential oil is only one of many ways in which a plant can be prepared as a remedy. German chamomile, for example, is used extensively as a herbal preparation, as well as being utilized for its volatile oil. It is important to distinguish between an oil's therapeutic qualities and those of the herb taken as a whole. Peppermint oil, for example, is used to treat respiratory conditions as an inhalant, because of its antispasmodic and antiseptic action. But for the longer-term treatment of digestive disorders it is better to use extracts from the whole herb, where the action of the volatile oil is supported by the presence of bitters and tannins.

FRESH CHAMOMILE

FRESH PEPPERMINT

FRESH YARROW

In 1964, French doctor and scientist Dr. Jean Valnet used essential oils as part of a program by which he successfully treated specific medical and psychiatric disorders, the results of which were published in the book *Aromatherapie*.

The work of Valnet was studied by Madame Marguerite Maury, who applied his research to her beauty therapy, in which she attempted to revitalize her clients by creating a strictly personal aromatic complex that she tried to adapt to the temperament and particular health problems of each subject.

In many ways "aromatherapy" is a misleading term, suggesting that it is a form of healing that works exclusively through the sense of smell, and on the emotions. In addition to its scent, each essential oil has an individual combination of constituents that interact with the body's chemistry in a direct manner, which then in turn affects certain organs or systems as a whole. For example, when the oils are used externally in the form of a massage treatment, they are easily absorbed through the skin and transported throughout the body. This can be

## MADAME MARGUERITE MAURY

Marguerite Maury (1895–1968) was a dedicated and inspired woman who did much to establish the reputation of aromatherapy. She set up the first aromatherapy clinics in France, Britain, and Switzerland and was awarded two international prizes (in 1962 and 1967 respectively) for her studies on essential oils and cosmetology. She focused on the rejuvenating properties of essential oils in her research work, the results of which were published in English as *The Secret of Life and Youth* (1964).

Odor signals are passed *directly* to the limbic system of the brain, evoking an *immediate* emotional or instinctual response.

Aromatic molecules enter the *lungs* and are absorbed via the alveoli into the blood.

The blood is carried to the *heart* and transported throughout the body via the circulatory system.

Different oils have affinities with specific parts of the body – e.g. spices particularly affect the *digestion*.

Waste and toxins are processed by the *liver and kidneys* and eliminated mainly via the lungs, but also in the urine and sweat.

demonstrated by rubbing a clove of garlic on the soles of the feet; the volatile oil content will be taken into the blood and the odor will appear on the breath a little while later.

Essential oils have three distinct modes of action in interrelating with the human body: pharmacological, physiological, and psychological. The pharmacological effect relates to the chemical changes that take place when an essential oil enters the bloodstream and reacts with hormones, enzymes, and so on. The physiological mode is concerned with the way in which an essential oil affects body systems. The psychological effect takes place when an essence is inhaled and an individual responds to its odor.

RIGHT *Airborne aromatic oil molecules interact with the different body systems. Some oils are noted for their particular affinities to specific body systems.*

# How Essential Oils Work

THE THERAPEUTIC POTENTIAL *of essential oils, like other plant-derived remedies, has yet to be fully realized. Although numerous medical herbs have been utilized since antiquity, many of which have been exploited to provide the biologically active compounds that form the basis of most of our modern drugs, there is still a great deal to be learned about their precise pharmacology. This is particularly true of aromatic oils, which have a concentrated yet multifaceted makeup. Modern research has largely confirmed the traditionally held beliefs regarding the therapeutic uses of particular plants. Like herbal remedies, an essential oil can cover a wide field of activities; the same herb or oil can stimulate certain systems of the body while sedating or relaxing others. In order to gain a clearer understanding of the way essential oils work, and some of their particular areas of activity, it may be helpful to take an overall view of the systems of the human body.*

## THE SKIN

Skin problems are often the surface manifestation of deeper conditions, such as buildup of toxins in the blood, hormonal imbalance, or nervous and emotional difficulties. Versatile essential oils are able to combat such complaints on a variety of levels. Since essential oils are soluble in oil and alcohol and impart their scent to water, they are an ideal ingredient for cosmetics and skin care as well as for the treatment of specific diseases.

### ANTISEPTICS

for cuts, insect bites, blemishes, etc.; for example, thyme, sage, eucalyptus, tea tree, clove, lavender, lemon.

### ANTI-INFLAMMATORY

for eczema, infected wounds, bumps, bruises, etc.; for example, German and Roman chamomile, lavender, yarrow.

### FUNGICIDAL OILS

for athlete's foot, candida, ringworm, etc.; for example, lavender, tea tree, myrrh, patchouli, sweet marjoram.

### GRANULATION STIMULATING OR CICATRIZING (HEALING) AGENTS

for burns, cuts and scars, stretch marks, etc.; for example, lavender, chamomile, rose, orange blossom, frankincense, geranium.

### DEODORANTS

for excessive perspiration, cleaning wounds, etc.; for example, bergamot, lavender, thyme, juniper, cypress, Spanish sage, lemongrass.

### INSECT REPELLENTS AND PARASITICIDES

for lice, fleas, scabies, ticks, mosquitoes, ants, moths, etc.; for example, spike lavender, garlic, geranium, citronella, eucalyptus, clove, camphor, Atlas cedarwood.

FRESH SPIKE LAVENDER

FRESH SWEET MARJORAM

## THE CIRCULATION, MUSCLES, AND JOINTS

Essential oils are easily absorbed via the skin and mucosa into the bloodstream, affecting the nature of the circulation as a whole. Oils with a rubefacient or warming effect, such as black pepper, camphor, and sweet marjoram, not only cause better local blood circulation but also influence the inner organs. They bring a warmth and glow to the surface of the skin and can provide considerable pain relief through their analgesic or numbing effect. Such oils can also relieve local inflammation by setting free mediators in the body which in turn cause the blood vessels to expand, so the blood is able to move more quickly and the swelling is reduced. Some oils, such as hyssop, tend to have a balancing or regulating effect on the circulatory system as a whole, reducing the blood pressure if it is too high or stimulating the system if it is sluggish.

### HYPOTENSIVES

for high blood pressure, palpitations, stress, etc.;
for example, sweet marjoram, ylang ylang, lavender, lemon.

### HYPERTENSIVES

for poor circulation, chilblains, listlessness, etc.; for example,
rosemary, spike lavender, eucalyptus, peppermint, thyme.

### RUBEFACIENTS

for rheumatism of the joints, muscular stiffness, sciatica,
lumbago, etc.; for example, black pepper, juniper, rosemary,
camphor, sweet marjoram.

### DEPURATIVE OR ANTITOXIC AGENTS

for arthritis, gout, congestion, skin eruptions, etc.;
for example, juniper, lemon, fennel, lovage.

### LYMPHATIC STIMULANTS

for cellulitis, obesity, water retention, etc.; for example,
grapefruit, lime, fennel, lemon, mandarin, white birch.

### CIRCULATORY TONICS AND ASTRINGENTS

for swellings, inflammations, varicose veins, etc.;
for example, cypress, yarrow, lemon.

FRESH JUNIPER

FRESH PEPPERMINT

FRESH LOVAGE

FRESH CYPRESS

FRESH LEMON

FRESH FENNEL

## THE RESPIRATORY SYSTEM

Nose, throat, and lung infections are conditions that respond very well to treatment with essential oils. Inhalation is a very effective way of utilizing their properties; they are absorbed into the blood circulation even faster than by oral application. Most essential oils that are absorbed from the stomach are then excreted via the lungs.

FRESH TOLU BALSUM

## THE DIGESTIVE SYSTEM

Although it is not recommended that essential oils be taken orally, they can effect certain changes in the digestive processes by external application. Herbal remedies for digestive complaints combine aromatic components with bitters, tannins, and mucilage, which are absent in the volatile oil alone. The external application of essential oils is consequently somewhat limited compared with the internal use of herbal remedies.

FRESH SWEET ORANGE

### EXPECTORANTS

for catarrh, sinusitis, coughs, bronchitis, etc.; for example, eucalyptus, pine, thyme, myrrh, sandalwood, fennel.

### ANTISPASMODICS

for colic, asthma, dry cough, whooping cough, etc.; for example, hyssop, cypress, Atlas cedarwood, bergamot, chamomile, cajeput.

### BALSAMIC AGENTS

for colds, chills, congestion, etc.; for example, benzoin, frankincense, Tolu balsam, Peru balsam, myrrh.

### ANTISEPTICS

for flu, colds, sore throat, tonsillitis, gingivitis, etc.; for example, thyme, sage, eucalyptus, hyssop, pine, cajeput, tea tree, borneol.

FRESH HYSSOP

### ANTISPASMODICS

for spasm, pain, indigestion, etc.; for example, chamomile, caraway, fennel, orange, peppermint, lemon balm, aniseed, cinnamon.

### CARMINATIVES AND STOMACHICS

for flatulent dyspepsia, aerophagia, nausea, etc.; for example, angelica, basil, fennel, chamomile, peppermint, mandarin.

### CHOLAGOGUES

for increasing the flow of bile and stimulating the gall bladder; for example, caraway, lavender, peppermint, borneol.

### HEPATICS

for liver congestions, jaundice, etc.; for example, lemon, lime, rosemary, peppermint.

### APERITIFS

for loss of appetite, anorexia, etc.; for example, aniseed, angelica, orange, ginger, garlic.

FRESH COMMON SAGE

GARLIC

FRESH BASIL

## GENITOURINARY/ ENDOCRINE SYSTEMS

The reproductive system can be affected by absorption via the skin into the bloodstream, as well as through hormonal changes. Some essential oils such as rose and jasmine have an affinity for the reproductive system. They have a strengthening effect and also help to combat specific complaints such as menstrual problems, genital infections, and sexual difficulties. Some oils, such as hops, sage and fennel contain plant oils that mimic corresponding human hormones, such as estrogen. Other essential oils are known to influence the levels of hormone secretion of other glands, including the thyroid gland, adrenal medulla, and adrenal cortex.

FRESH BERGAMOT

FRESH ROSE
PETALS

FENNEL LEAVES
AND SEEDS

FRESH JASMINE

FRESH SWEET
MARJORAM

MYRRH

BLACK
PEPPERCORNS

GERANIUM

### ANTISPASMODICS

for menstrual cramp (dysmenorrhea), labor pains, etc.; for example, sweet marjoram, chamomile, clary sage, jasmine, lavender.

### EMMENAGOGUES

for scanty periods, lack of periods (amenorrhea), etc.; for example, chamomile, fennel, hyssop, juniper, sweet marjoram, peppermint.

### UTERINE TONICS AND REGULATORS

for pregnancy, excess menstruation (menorrhagia), PMS, etc.; for example, clary sage, jasmine, rose, myrrh, frankincense, lemon balm.

### ANTISEPTIC AND BACTERICIDAL AGENTS

for leucorrhea, vaginal pruritis, thrush, etc.; for example, bergamot, chamomile, myrrh, rose, tea tree.

### GALACTAGOGUES

for increasing milk flow; for example, fennel, jasmine, anise, lemongrass (sage, mint, and parsley reduce it).

### APHRODISIACS

for impotence and frigidity, etc.; for example, black pepper, cardomon, clary sage, orange blossom, jasmine, rose, sandalwood, patchouli, ylang ylang.

### ANAPHRODISIACS

for reducing sexual desire; for example, sweet marjoram, camphor.

### ADRENAL STIMULANTS

for anxiety, stress-related conditions, etc.; for example, basil, geranium, rosemary, borneol, sage, pine, savory.

### URINARY ANTISEPTICS

for cystitis, urethritis, etc.; for example, bergamot, chamomile, tea tree, sandalwood.

## THE IMMUNE SYSTEM

Virtually all essential oils have bactericidal properties, and by promoting the production of white blood cells they can help prevent and treat infectious illness. It is these properties that gave aromatic herbs and oils such high repute with regard to infections such as malaria and typhoid in the tropics and epidemics of plague in the Middle Ages. "People who use essential oils all the time … mostly have a high level of resistance to illness, catching fewer colds etc., than average and recovering quickly if they do."[1]

FRESH LAVENDER LEAVES

## THE NERVOUS SYSTEM

Research shows that the properties of many oils correspond to the traditionally held views: chamomile, bergamot, and sandalwood were found to have a sedative effect on the central nervous system; jasmine and clove were stimulating. Some oils are known to be "adaptogens," that is, they have a balancing or normalizing effect on the systems of the body. Words like "relaxing" and "uplifting" often relate more to odor description and emotional response than physiological effect, although the two are related.

### BACTERIAL AND ANTIVIRAL AGENTS (PROPHYLACTICS)

for protection against colds, flu, etc.; for example, tea tree, cajeput, niaouli, basil, lavender, eucalyptus, bergamot, camphor, clove, rosemary.

### FEBRIFUGE AGENTS

for reducing fever and temperature, etc.; for example, angelica, basil, peppermint, thyme, sage, lemon, eucalyptus, tea tree.

### SUDORIFICS AND DIAPHORETICS

for promoting sweating, eliminating toxins, etc.; for example, rosemary, thyme, hyssop, chamomile.

### SEDATIVES

for nervous tensions, stress, insomnia, etc.; for example, chamomile, bergamot, sandalwood, lavender, sweet marjoram, lemon balm, hops, valerian, lemon.

### STIMULANTS

for convalescence, lack of strength, nervous fatigue, etc.; for example, basil, jasmine, peppermint, ylang ylang, orange blossom, angelica, rosemary.

### NERVE TONICS

for strengthening the nervous system as a whole; for example, chamomile, clary sage, juniper, lavender, marjoram, rosemary.

SLICED ANGELICA ROOT

FRESH BASIL

FRESH HYSSOP

FRESH NIAOULI

LEFT *These essential oils have been used to prevent and treat infectious diseases since the Middle Ages. Lavender is also used to strengthen the nervous system as a whole, while basil is known to have a stimulating effect on the central nervous system.*

## THE MIND

This is perhaps the most discussed and yet least understood area of activity regarding essential oils. There is no doubt that throughout history aromatic oils have been used for their power to influence the emotions and states of mind: this is the basis for their use as incense for religious and ritualistic purposes.

Recent research in England and Japan has aimed to put traditionally held beliefs into a scientific context. Two types of reactions to odors have been identified: a "hard-wired" response that is instinctual and ingrained from birth, and a "soft-wired" response that is learned or acquired later on.

But to what extent is the effect of a particular oil dependent upon its chemical or physiological make-up, and to what extent does it rely upon a belief or an association? In dealing with the psychological or emotional responses to the scent of a particular oil, it is appropriate to consider the temperament of each individual, rather than predict a set reaction. The effect of an odor on a human being is dependent upon the circumstances in which it is applied, the type of person, his or her mood, and previous associations.

At the Psychology of Perfumery conference 1991, it was generally agreed that "while pharmacological effects may be very similar from one person to another, psychological effects are bound to be different." The effect of an odor on a human being is dependent on a variety of factors, which include:

**1** *How the odor was applied.*
**2** *How much was applied.*
**3** *The circumstances in which it was applied.*
**4** *The person to whom it was applied (age, sex, personality type).*
**5** *What mood they were in to start with.*
**6** *What previous associations they may have with the odor.*
**7** *Anosmia, or inability to smell (certain scents).*

When we begin to consider individual needs, essential oils start to demonstrate the versatility of their nature. The rose is a good example of this: a flower associated with beauty, love, and spiritual depth in folklore and religious texts, but also with a long tradition of usage for physical conditions such as skin problems, regulating the female cycle, promoting the circulation, purifying the blood, and as a heart tonic. When we smell the fragrance of the rose, it carries all these rich associations with it, affecting our mind and body simultaneously, as the effect is molded by personal experience.

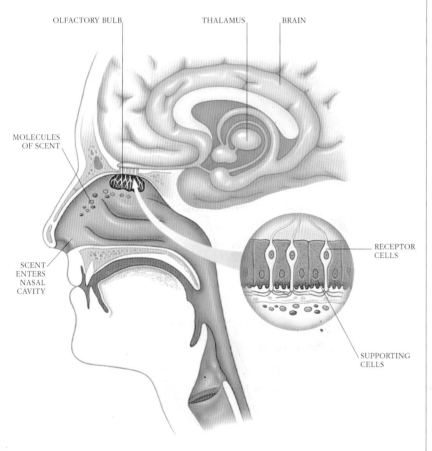

OLFACTORY BULB    THALAMUS    BRAIN

MOLECULES OF SCENT

SCENT ENTERS NASAL CAVITY

RECEPTOR CELLS

SUPPORTING CELLS

ABOVE *Two olfactory nerve tracts run right into the limbic system (the part of the brain concerned with memory and motion), which means that scents can evoke an immediate and powerful response that defies rational analysis.*

# How to Use Essential Oils in the Home

ESSENTIAL OILS CAN BE USED *at home in a variety of ways. They can be used as perfumes and to revive potpourris; they can be added to the bath and used to make individual beauty preparations. They can also be employed in the treatment of minor first-aid cases and to help prevent and relieve many common complaints such as headaches, colds, period pains, and aching muscles.*

## MASSAGE

Professional aromatherapists choose specific essential oils to suit the condition and temperament of the patient, which are then blended with a base oil, such as sweet almond oil. The essential oil content in a blend should usually be between 1 per cent and 3 per cent, depending on the type of disorder. Physical ailments such as

LEFT *A few drops of essential oil added to dried flower petals and seed-heads makes a fragrant pot-pourri.*

### R E C I P E

| ESSENTIAL OIL | BASE OIL |
|---|---|
| 20 to 60 drops | 3½fl oz (100ml) |
| 7 to 25 drops | 1fl oz (25ml) |
| 3 to 5 drops | 1 tsp (5ml) |

## STEP BY STEP MASSAGE

### EFFLEURAGE (STROKING MOVEMENTS)
*Make sure hands and oil are warm. Use slow, rhythmic strokes to rub the oil well into the skin, keeping the hands in contact with the body.*

### PETRISSAGE (KNEADING MOVEMENTS)
*Suitable for areas of muscular tightness or tension. Use a gentle kneading movement to squeeze and roll the surface skin together with the layers beneath.*

### FRICTION (CIRCULAR MOVEMENTS)
*Especially beneficial for areas of cold, numbness, and poor circulation. Rub the skin in a vigorous circular movement with the flat palms of the hand.*

rheumatism demand a stronger concentration than more emotional or nervous conditions. Massage is a relaxing and nourishing experience in itself, and ensures that the oils are effectively absorbed through the skin into the bloodstream.

## SKIN OILS AND LOTIONS

The essential oils are prepared much as they would be for a massage, except that the base oil should include the more nourishing oils such as jojoba, avocado, or apricot kernel oil. A gentle circular movement of the fingers is often enough for the oils to be absorbed. Rose and neroli are good for dry or

LEFT *Since ancient times, perfumes and cosmetics have been used to enhance appearance.*

## HOT AND COLD COMPRESSES

This is an effective way of using essential oils to relieve pain such as backache, rheumatism, earache, and toothache. Fill a bowl with very hot water, then add 4 or 5 drops of essential oil. Dip a folded piece of cloth, absorbent cotton, or a face cloth into the bowl, squeeze out excess water, and place on the affected area.

mature complexions; geranium, bergamot, and lemon can help combat acne and greasy skin.

---

### DIFFERENT SKIN TYPES

#### OILY SKIN

Oily skin is prone to congestion, often resulting in blemishes and blackheads. Hygiene is very important, but care should be taken not to disturb the natural pH balance of the skin. Astringent and antiseptic essential oils are indicated, such as tea tree bergamot, or geranium. Generally, the base oils should be kept light so that they can be absorbed easily – apricot kernel, peach kernel, or jojoba are ideal.

#### DRY SKIN

A dry complexion becomes wrinkled more easily than oily skin, especially if it is exposed to too much sun or the effects of central heating. It therefore needs to be moisturized thoroughly and regularly. Dry skin also often tends to be sensitive, so mild essences such as sandalwood, chamomile, and rose are indicated. Rich, nourishing base oils, like hazelnut, avocado, and evening primrose oils, are valuable hydrating agents.

#### MATURE SKIN

Aging is inevitable, but essential oils can do much to slow down the effects. The regular use of facial treatments containing cytophylactic oils (those that stimulate new cell growth and prevent wrinkles) is vital – such oils include lavender, neroli, and frankincense. Base oils rich in Vitamin E, notably borage and wheatgerm, are especially beneficial for promoting cell regeneration; rosehip seed oil is also indicated.

TRUE LAVENDER

ROSE PETALS

GERANIUM

## HAIR CARE

The hair can be enhanced by the use of a few drops of essential oils in the final hair rinse or added straight to a mild shampoo. Oils such as rosemary, West Indian bay, and chamomile all help to condition and encourage healthy hair growth.

RIGHT *An aromatic diffuser with a ribbon wick vaporizes the oil and disperses the scent through the room.*

### RECIPE

#### ALCOHOL-BASED SCALP RUB

This alcohol-based scalp rub can be used to condition the hair or to get rid of unwanted parasites such as lice and fleas. Add 1 tsp (5ml) of essential oil to 3½fl oz (100ml) of vodka.

#### CONDITIONING TREATMENT

Add about 3 per cent of an essential oil to a base oil such as olive oil with jojoba or sweet almond oil and massage into the scalp, then wrap the head in warm towels for an hour or two.

DRIED
ROSE
BUDS

## FLOWER WATER

It is possible to make toilet or flower water at home by adding about 20 to 30 drops of essential oil to a 3½ fl oz (100 ml) bottled spring or de-ionized water, leaving it for a few days in the dark and then filtering it using a coffee filter paper. This method can be very helpful in the prevention and treatment of skin conditions such as acne, dermatitis, and eczema, and to tone and cleanse the complexion. Traditional oils include rose, orange blossom, lavender, and petitgrain.

## DOUCHE

In the case of candida or thrush, add between 5 and 10 drops of tea tree to 1¾ pints (1 liter) of warm water and shake well. This mixture can be used on a sitz bath, bidet, or put into an enema/douche pot.

## VAPORIZATION

Scent a room with an oil burner or aromatic diffuser. Alternatively, a few drops of oil can be placed on a light bulb ring or added to a small bowl of water placed on a radiator. Frankincense and cedarwood create a peaceful and relaxed mood.

DRIED ROMAN
CHAMOMILE

ORANGE BLOSSOM LEAVES

ROSEMARY

LAVENDER

## STEAM INHALATION

Especially suited to sinus, throat, and chest infections. Add about 5 drops of an oil such as peppermint or thyme to a bowl of hot water, cover the head and bowl with a towel and breathe deeply for a minute – then repeat. Sitting in a steaming hot bath is another way of inhaling a certain amount of essential oil. Oils such as lemon or tea tree can help to unclog the pores and clear the complexion.

## BATHS

Add 5 or 10 drops of oil to the bathwater when the tub is full. Aromatic bathing treats a wide range of complaints, including irritated skin conditions, muscular aches and pains, rheumatism and arthritis.

## NEAT APPLICATION

Generally speaking, essential oils are not applied to the skin in an undiluted form. However, lavender, for example, can be applied to burns, cuts, and insect bites. Certain oils, such as jasmine and rose, make excellent perfumes.

ORANGE BLOSSOM

### CAUTION

**Internal use**: due to the high concentration of essential oils, it is not recommended that they be taken at home in this manner. Since essential oils are readily absorbed through the skin, they can affect the internal organs by external use.

BELOW *"The Bath" by Alfred George Stevens. Aromatic bathing can relieve stress-related complaints, such as anxiety and insomnia, and aches and pains.*

# Creative Blending

ESSENTIAL OILS ARE BLENDED *for two reasons: for their therapeutic effects on a physical condition such as backache; or to create a perfume, which stimulates an emotional or esthetic response. A person who is suffering from a physical complaint also has a psychic or emotional disposition, which will naturally respond in a more subtle way to a particular blend of oils. Similarly, a personal perfume that expresses the unique personality of an individual through fragrance has a generally remedial effect on the person as a whole.*

## CORRECT PROPORTIONS

For therapeutic purposes, essential oils are usually diluted before being applied to the skin. To make a massage or body oil, the essential oil or oils should first be mixed with a light base oil such as grapeseed or sweet almond oil. The essential oil content in a blend is usually between 1 and 3 per cent. Physical ailments demand a stronger concentration of essential oils than emotional or nervous conditions.

RIGHT *Correct proportions are important in blending essential oils, as are individual perfume preferences. Some scents can be incompatible – a floral blend, for example, would be unacceptable to most men.*

---

### A SIMPLE BLENDING GUIDE

Each essential oil blends well with members of its own family or group, or with members from a neighboring group, e.g. Citrus and Floral, or Spicy and Woody.

*GROUP A:* WOODY
e.g. cedarwood and pine

*GROUP B:* HERBACEOUS
e.g. rosemary and clary sage

*GROUP C:* CITRUS
e.g. bergamot and lemon

*GROUP D:* FLORAL
e.g. geranium and rose

*GROUP E:* RESINOUS
e.g. galbanum and frankincense

*GROUP F:* SPICY
e.g. ginger and black pepper

RIGHT *The exotic perfume "Shalimar" by Guerlain is dominated by woody or musky oils. It contains Peru balsam, benzoin, opopanax, vanilla, patchouli, rose, jasmine, orris, vetvier, rosewood, lemon, bergamot, and mandarin.*

## SYNERGIES

Some oils blended together have a mutually enhancing effect upon one another. In general, oils of the same botanical family blend well together, as do those that share common constituents, such as the camphoraceous oils. Some oils, such as rose, jasmine, oakmoss, and lavender, enhance just about any blend.

## PERSONAL PERFUMES

An individual fragrance needs the correct balance of color or flavors, and also generally has a theme. A perfume should have a focus around which the other fragrances unite. The overall character of a perfume also benefits from unusual or diverse combinations that can give it character.

ABOVE *"The Perfume Makers" by Albert Sorkau presents an idealized portrait of the nineteenth-century perfume industry.*

## PIESSE'S LEGACY

In the nineteenth century, a Frenchman named Piesse classified odors according to the notes in a musical scale. The following list provides a general idea of the dominant character of selected oils.

### TOP NOTES
A fresh, light, immediate quality
e.g. eucalyptus, lemon, basil

### MIDDLE NOTES
The heart of the fragrance
e.g. geranium, lavender, marjoram

### BASE NOTES
A rich, heavy, lingering scent
e.g. patchouli, jasmine, myrrh

A well-balanced perfume is said to contain elements from each of these different categories, the quantities of each determining whether it is a heavy oriental-type scent or a light, floral aroma.

# A Guide to Aromatic Materials

OVER THIRTY FAMILIES OF PLANTS, *with about ninety species, represent the main oil-producing group. The majority of spices originate in tropical countries; conversely, the majority of herbs are grown in temperate climates. The same plant grown in a different region and under different conditions can produce essential oils of widely diverse characteristics, which are known as "chemotypes." Common thyme* (Thymus vulgaris)*, for example, produces several chemotypes depending on its growth conditions and dominant constituent, notably the citral or linalol types, the thyuanol type, and the thymol or carvacrol type. It is important to know not only the botanical name of the plant from which the oil has been produced, but also its place of origin and main constituents. One of the principal ways of defining the qualities of a particular oil and checking its purity is to ascertain the specific blend of components and to look at its chemical character.*

RIGHT *An herb garden with a chamomile path. Most herbs grow in temperate climates, whereas the majority of spices come from tropical climates.*

# CHEMISTRY

In general, essential oils consist of chemical compounds that have hydrogen, carbon, and oxygen as their building blocks. These can be subdivided into two groups: the hydrocarbons, which are made up almost exclusively of terpenes (monoterpenes, sesquiterpenes, and diterpenes); and the oxygenated compounds, mainly esters, aldehydes, ketones, alcohols, phenols, and oxides; acids, lactones, sulfur, and nitrogen compounds are sometimes also present.

## TERPENES

Common terpene hydrocarbons include limonene (antiviral, found in 90 per cent of citrus oils) and pinene (antiseptic, found in high proportions in pine and turpentine oils); also camphene, cadinene, caryophyllene, cedrene, dipentene, phellandrene, terpinene, sabinene, and myrcene among others. Sesquiterpenes have outstanding anti-inflammatory and bactericidal properties.

GRAPEFRUIT PEEL, LEAF, AND YOUNG FRUIT

## ESTERS

Probably the most widespread group found in essential oils, which includes linalyl acetate (found in bergamot, clary sage, and lavender) and geranyl acetate (found in sweet marjoram). They are characteristically fungicidal and sedative, often having a fruity aroma. Other esters include bornyl acetate, eugenyl acetate, and lavendulyl acetate.

## ALDEHYDES

Citral, citronellal, and neural are important aldehydes found notably in lemon-scented oils such as melissa, lemongrass, lemon verbena, citronella, etc. Aldehydes in general have a sedative effect; citral has antiseptic properties. Other aldehydes include benzaldehyde, cinnamic aldehyde, cuminic aldehyde, and perillaldehyde.

FRESH PENNYROYAL

## KETONES

Some of the most common toxic constituents are ketones, such as thujone found in mugwort, tansy, sage and wormwood; and pulegone found in pennyroyal and buchu. Nontoxic ketones include jasmone (in jasmine) and fenchone (in fennel oil). Other ketones include camphor, carvone, methone, and pinocamphone.

FRESH SPIKE LAVENDER

## ALCOHOLS

These compounds have good antiseptic and antiviral properties with an uplifting quality; they are also generally nontoxic. Among the most common terpene alcohols are linalol ( in rosewood, linaloe, and lavender), citronellol (in rose, lemon, eucalyptus and geranium) and geraniol (found in palmarosa); also borneol, methol, terpineol, nerol, farnesol, vetiverol, benzyl alcohol, and cedrol.

## PHENOLS

These tend to have a bactericidal and strongly stimulating effect, but can be skin irritants. Common phenols include eugenol (found in clove and West Indian bay), thymol (found in thyme), carvacrol (found in oregano and savory); also methyl eugenol, methyl chavicol, anethole, safrole, myristicin, and apiol among others.

FRESH SUMMER SAVORY

## OXIDES

By far the most important oxide is cineol (or eucalyptol). It has an expectorant effect, well known as the principal constituent of eucalyptus oil. It is also found in a wide range of other oils, especially those of a camphoraceous nature such as rosemary, bay laurel, tea tree, and cajeput. Other oxides include linalol oxide found in hyssop (decumbent variety), ascaridol, bisabolol oxide, and bisabolone oxide.

FRESH BAY LEAVES

FRESH ROSEMARY

# Methods of Extraction

THE TERM "ESSENTIAL OIL" *is loosely applied to all aromatic products or extracts that are derived from natural sources. This is not strictly accurate, since many fragrance products, although they are used by the perfumery industry, are only partially composed of essential oils. The terms "concrete", "absolute", and "resinoid" should be used to denote a type of product that contains a mixture of volatile and nonvolatile components, such as wax or resin, but in the marketplace this is often not the case. Some plant materials, especially flowers, are subject to deterioration and should be processed as soon as possible after harvesting; others, including seeds and roots, are stored or transported for extraction. The extraction method used depends on the quality of the material being used and the type of aromatic product that is required.*

## ESSENTIAL OILS

An essential oil is extracted from the plant material by two main methods: by simple expression or pressure, as is the case with most of the citrus oils; or by steam, water, or dry distillation. The majority of oils are produced by distillation. This process isolates only the volatile and water-insoluble parts of the plant – many other constituents are consequently excluded.

EUCALYPTUS BARK

FRESH SCHINUS MOLLE LEAVES

FRESH DILL

ABOVE *This type of apparatus, with a false bottom, was used for the distillation of plants such as peppermint and lavender.*

## CONCRETES

Concretes are prepared almost exclusively from raw materials of vegetable origin, such as the bark, flower, leaf, herb, or root. The aromatic plant material is subjected to extraction by hydrocarbon-type solvents, rather than distillation or expression. This is necessary when the essential oil is adversely affected by hot water and steam, as is the case with jasmine. It also produces a more true-to-nature fragrance.

ORRIS ROOT

MARIGOLD FLOWER

## RESINOIDS

Resinoids are prepared from natural resinous material by extraction with a hydrocarbon solvent, such as petroleum or hexane. Typical resinous materials are balsams (Peru balsam), resins (amber), oleoresins (turpentine), and oleo gum resins (myrrh). They can be viscous liquids, semisolid, or solid, but are usually homogenous masses of noncrystalline character.

PERU BALSAM
LEAVES

## ABSOLUTES

An absolute is obtained from the concrete by a second process of solvent extraction, using pure alcohol in which the unwanted wax is only slightly soluble. A further process of molecular distillation can be used to remove every last trace of nonvolatile matter. The alcohol is recovered by evaporation, which requires a gentle vacuum towards the end of the process.

FRESH CLARY
SAGE

*RIGHT True pomades are the products of a process known as enfleurage, in which a layer of fat is saturated with fragrance from cut flowers. This process is virtually obsolete today.*

FRESH MASTIC

## POMADES

Pomades were made by placing a coating of odorless fat on glass. Freshly cut flowers, laid on the fat, saturated it with their volatile oils. The fat was then treated with alcohol to produce pure absolutes.

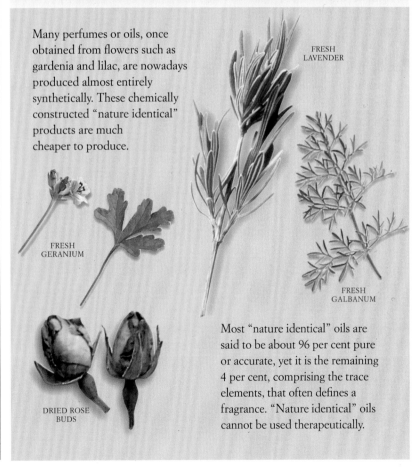

## NATURAL VERSUS "NATURE IDENTICAL"

Many perfumes or oils, once obtained from flowers such as gardenia and lilac, are nowadays produced almost entirely synthetically. These chemically constructed "nature identical" products are much cheaper to produce.

FRESH
LAVENDER

FRESH
GERANIUM

FRESH
GALBANUM

DRIED ROSE
BUDS

Most "nature identical" oils are said to be about 96 per cent pure or accurate, yet it is the remaining 4 per cent, comprising the trace elements, that often defines a fragrance. "Nature identical" oils cannot be used therapeutically.

# Therapeutic Index

ESSENTIAL OILS CAN BE USED *to treat a wide range of common complaints, including those listed on the following pages. Special care must be taken regarding the use of oils that can cause irritation in concentration, and oils known to be phototoxic, such as bergamot and lemon. Before using a particular oil, consult the Safety Guidelines. Many of the conditions mentioned in the following pages could benefit from aromatherapy used with other forms of treatment, such as diet, exercise, and herbal medicine.*

## ABBREVIATED TERMS USED IN THIS SECTION

| | | | |
|---|---|---|---|
| **B** | BATH | **I** | INHALATION (*STEAM*) |
| **C** | COMPRESS | **M** | MASSAGE |
| **D** | DOUCHE | **N** | NEAT APPLICATION |
| **F** | FLOWER WATER | **S** | SKIN OIL/LOTION |
| **H** | HAIR CARE | **V** | VAPORIZATION |

In the following pages common complaints are grouped according to different parts of the body: Skin Care; Circulation, Muscles, and Joints; Respiratory System; Digestive System; Genitourinary and Endocrine Systems; Immune System; Nervous System. The table above is a guide to abbreviated terms of suggested application, found throughout the Index pages.

## THERAPEUTIC GUIDELINES

As a general rule that is in line with the present-day aromatherapy "code of practice", it is best to use essential oils as external remedies only. This is due to the high concentration of the oils and the potential irritation or damage that they can cause to the mucous membranes and delicate stomach lining in undiluted form. There even seems to be some kind of natural order in this scheme, in that volatile oils mix readily with oils and ointments suited to external application, which are absorbed readily through the skin and vaporize easily for inhalation. When inhaled, they can have an effect on the individual's mood or feelings, at the same time causing physiological changes in the body.

These are only superficial guidelines, for there are always exceptions to the rule. Plantain, for example, is an excellent wound-healing herb valuable for external use, although it does not contain any essential oil. Nor can we ignore the fact that a great many aromatic oils are used for flavoring our food and beverages and are consumed daily in minute amounts. For example, peppermint oil is used in a wide variety of alcoholic and non-alcoholic beverages, confectionery, and prepared savory foods, although the highest average use does not exceed 0.104 per cent. Mint oils are used extensively by the pharmaceutical industry in products such as toothpaste, cough and cold remedies, and by the cosmetic industry in soaps, creams, lotions, colognes, and perfumes.

The use of essential oils covers a wide and varied spectrum. On the one hand, they share the holistic qualities of natural plant remedies. On the other hand, they play an active role in the pharmaceutical industry, either in their entirety or in the form of isolated constituents such as "phenol" or "menthol".

It is not the aim of this book to glorify natural remedies (some of which are in fact highly toxic) at the expense of scientific progress, nor to uphold the principles of our drug-oriented culture, but simply to provide information about the multifaceted oils themselves.

### CAUTION

**Babies and children:** Always increase the dilution for babies and infants to at least half the recommended amount. For babies, avoid the possibly toxic and irritant oils altogether.

## SAFETY GUIDELINES

### HAZARDOUS OILS
Some oils have high toxicity levels or can cause dermal irritation. Avoid bitter almond, arnica, boldo, broom, buchu, calamus, camphor (brown and yellow), cassia, chervil, cinnamon (bark), costus, deertongue, elecampane, fennel (bitter), horseradish, jaborandi, melilotus, mugwort, mustard, oregano, pennyroyal, pine (dwarf), rue, sage (common), santolina, sassafras, savine, savory, tansy, thuja, thyme (red), tonka, wintergreen, wormseed, and wormwood.

LOVAGE SPRIG

### TOXICITY
The following oils should be used in moderation (only in dilution and for a maximum of two weeks at a time): aniseed, basil (exotic), bay laurel, bay (West Indian), calamintha, camphor (white), cascarrilla bark, cassie, cedarwood (Virginian), cinnamon (leaf), clove (bud), cilantro, eucalyptus, fennel (sweet), hops, hyssop, juniper, nutmeg, parsley, pepper (black), sage (Spanish), tagetes, tarragon, thyme (white), tuberose, turmeric, turpentine, valerian.

### NEAT APPLICATION
In general, do not apply neat to skin – dilute in carrier oil or cream. Exceptions to this rule include lavender, ylang ylang, and sandalwood. Always do a patch test first, and avoid eyes.

### DERMAL/SKIN IRRITATION
Oils that may irritate the skin, especially if used in a high concentration, are: ajowan, allspice, aniseed, basil (sweet), black pepper, borneol, cajeput, caraway, cedarwood (Virginian), cinnamon (leaf), clove (bud), cornmint, eucalyptus, garlic, ginger, lemon, parsley, peppermint, pine needle (Scotch and longleaf), thyme (white), and turmeric. These oils should be used in half the usual recommended dilutions. Always mix them first in a base oil, cream, or gel before applying.

### SENSITIZATION
Some oils may cause skin irritation in people with very sensitive skins or can cause an allergic reaction. It is important for those with sensitive skins always to do a patch test before using a new oil to check for individual sensitization. Oils that may cause sensitization: basil (French), bay laurel, benzoin, cade, cananga, cedarwood (Virginian), chamomile (Roman and German), citronella, garlic, geranium, ginger, hops, jasmine, lemon, lemongrass, lemon balm (melissa), litsea cubeba, lovage, mastic, mint, orange, Peru balsam, pine (Scotch and longleaf), styrax, tea tree, thyme (white), Tolu balsam, turmeric, turpentine, valerian, vanilla, verbena, violet, yarrow, and ylang ylang.

CUBEBA SPRIG

### PHOTOTOXICITY
Do not use the following oils either neat or in dilution on the skin, if the area will be exposed to the sun: angelica root, bergamot (not bergapten-free type), cumin, ginger, lemon, lime, lovage, mandarin, orange, and verbena.

### PREGNANCY
During pregnancy, use essential oils in half the usual amount. Avoid the following: ajowan, angelica, anise star, aniseed, basil, bay laurel, calamintha, cedarwood (all types), celery seed, cinnamon leaf, citronella, clary sage, clove, cumin, fennel (sweet), hyssop, juniper, labdanum, lovage, marjoram, myrrh, nutmeg, parsley, snakeroot, Spanish sage, tarragon, and thyme (white). Avoid peppermint, rose, and rosemary in the first four months.

### HIGH BLOOD PRESSURE
Avoid the following in cases of high blood pressure (hypertension): hyssop, rosemary, sage (Spanish/common), thyme.

### EPILEPSY
Avoid the following in cases of epilepsy: fennel (sweet), hyssop, rosemary, and sage (all types).

### DIABETICS
Avoid angelica in cases of diabetes.

### HOMEOPATHY
Homeopathy is not compatible with black pepper, camphor, eucalyptus, and peppermint.

# Skin Care

## ACNE

Bergamot, camphor (white), cananga, cedarwood (Atlas, Texas, and Virginian), chamomile (German and Roman), clove bud, galbanum, geranium, grapefruit, helichrysum, juniper, lavandin, lavender (spike and true), lemon, lemongrass, lime, linaloe, litsea cubeba, mandarin, mint (peppermint and spearmint), myrtle, niaouli, palmarosa, patchouli, petitgrain, rosemary, rosewood, sage (clary and Spanish), sandalwood, tea tree, thyme, vetiver, violet, yarrow, ylang ylang.

*Suggested application:* **M S F B I N**

FRESH BERGAMOT

## ALLERGIES

Lemon balm, chamomile (German and Roman), helichrysum, true lavender, spikenard.

*Suggested application:* **M S F B I**

## ATHLETE'S FOOT

Clove bud, eucalyptus, lavender (spike and true), lemon, lemongrass, myrrh, patchouli, tea tree.

*Suggested application:* **S**

FRESH SPIKE LAVENDER

## BALDNESS AND HAIR CARE

West Indian bay, white birch, cedarwood (Atlas, Texas and Virginian), chamomile (German and Roman), grapefruit, juniper, patchouli, rosemary, sage (clary and Spanish), yarrow, ylang ylang.

*Suggested application:* **S H**

## BOILS, ABSCESSES, AND BLISTERS

Bergamot, chamomile (German and Roman), eucalyptus blue gum, galbanum, helichrysum, lavandin, lavender (spike and true), lemon, mastic, niaouli, clary sage, tea tree, thyme, turpentine.

*Suggested application:* **S C B**

## BRUISES

Arnica (cream), borneol, clove bud, fennel, geranium, hyssop, sweet marjoram, lavender, thyme.

*Suggested application:* **S C**

FRESH LEMON

## BURNS

Canadian balsam, chamomile (German and Roman), clove bud, eucalyptus blue gum, geranium, helichrysum, lavandin, lavender (spike and true), marigold, niaouli, tea tree, yarrow.

*Suggested application:* **C N**

MARIGOLD FLOWER

## CHAPPED AND CRACKED SKIN

Peru balsam, Tolu balsam, benzoin, myrrh, patchouli, sandalwood.

*Suggested application:* **S F B**

## CHILBLAINS

Chamomile (German and Roman), lemon, lime, sweet marjoram, black pepper.

*Suggested application:* **S N**

LEAVES AND FRUIT PEEL OF LIME

## COLD SORES/HERPES

Bergamot, eucalyptus blue gum, lemon, tea tree.
*Suggested application:* **S**

## CONGESTED AND DULL SKIN

Angelica, white birch, sweet fennel, geranium, grapefruit, lavandin, lavender (spike and true), lemon, lime, mandarin, mint (peppermint and spearmint), myrtle, niaouli, orange (bitter and sweet), palmarosa, rose (cabbage and damask), rosemary, rosewood, ylang ylang.
*Suggested application:* **M S F B I**

ROSE PETALS

## CUTS/SORES

Canadian balsam, benzoin, borneol, cabreuva, cade, chamomile (German and Roman), clove bud, elemi, eucalyptus (blue gum, lemon, and peppermint), galbanum, geranium, helichrysum, hyssop, lavandin, lavender (spike and true), lemon, lime, linaloe, marigold, mastic, myrrh, niaouli, Scotch pine, Spanish sage,
Levant styrax,
thyme, turpent
vetiver, yarrow.
*Suggested*
*application:*
**S C**

FRESH YARROW

## DANDRUFF

West Indian bay, cade, cedarwood (Atlas, Texas, and Virginian), eucalyptus, spike lavender,
lemon, patchouli, rosemary, sage
(clary and Spanish), tea tree.
*Suggested*
*application:*
**S H**

FRESH CADE

## DERMATITIS

White birch, cade, cananga, carrot seed, cedarwood (Atlas, Texas, and Virginian), chamomile (German and Roman), geranium, helichrysum, hops, hyssop, juniper, true lavender, linaloe, litsea cubeba, mint (peppermint and spearmint), palmarosa, patchouli, rosemary, sage (clary and Spanish), thyme. *Suggested application:* **M S C F B**

FRESH
VIRGINIAN
CEDARWOOD

## DRY AND SENSITIVE SKIN

Peru balsam, Tolu balsam, cassie, chamomile (German and Roman), frankincense, jasmine, lavandin, lavender (spike and true), rosewood, sandalwood, violet.
*Suggested application:* **M S F B**

## ECZEMA

Lemon balm, Peru balsam, Tolu balsam, bergamot, white birch, cade, carrot seed, cedarwood (Atlas, Texas, and Virginian), chamomile (German and Roman), geranium, helichrysum, hyssop,
juniper, lavandin, lavender

FRESH VIOLET

(spike and true), marigold, myrrh, patchouli, rose (cabbage and damask), rosemary, Spanish sage, thyme, violet, yarrow.
*Suggested application:*
**M S F B**

FRESH
PATCHOULI

## EXCESSIVE PERSPIRATION

Citronella, cypress, lemongrass, litsea cubeba, petitgrain, Scotch pine, Spanish sage.
*Suggested application:* **S B**

FRESH
CYPRESS

## GREASY OR OILY SKIN/SCALP

West Indian bay, bergamot, cajeput, camphor (white), cananga, carrot seed, citronella, cypress, sweet fennel, geranium, jasmine, juniper, lavender, lemon, lemongrass, litsea cubeba, mandarin, marigold, mimosa, myrtle, niaouli, palmarosa, patchouli, petitgrain, rosemary, rosewood, sandalwood, clary sage, tea tree, thyme, vetiver, ylang ylang.
*Suggested application:* **M S H F B**

FRESH FENNEL

## HEMORRHOIDS/PILES

Canadian balsam, copaiba balsam, cilantro, cubeb, cypress, geranium, juniper, myrrh, myrtle, parsley, yarrow.
*Suggested application:* **S C B**

## INSECT BITES

Lemon balm, French basil, bergamot, cajeput, cananga, chamomile (German and Roman), cinnamon leaf, blue gum eucalyptus, lavandin, lavender (spike and true), lemon, marigold, niaouli, tea tree, thyme, ylang ylang.
*Suggested application:* **S N**

FRESH CINNAMON

## INSECT REPELLENT

Lemon balm, French basil, bergamot, borneol, camphor (white), Virginian cedarwood, citronella, clove bud, cypress, eucalyptus (blue gum and lemon-scented), geranium, lavender, lemongrass, litsea cubeba, mastic, patchouli, rosemary, turpentine.
*Suggested application:* **S V**

FRESH MASTIC

## IRRITATED AND INFLAMED SKIN

Angelica, benzoin, camphor (white), Atlas cedarwood, chamomile (German and Roman), elemi, helichrysum, hyssop, jasmine, lavandin, true lavender, marigold, myrrh, patchouli, rose (cabbage and damask), clary sage, spikenard, tea tree, yarrow.
*Suggested application:* **S C F B**

DRIED ROSE BUDS

## LICE

Cinnamon leaf, blue gum eucalyptus, galbanum, geranium, lavandin, spike lavender, parsley, Scotch pine, rosemary, thyme, turpentine.
*Suggested application:* **S H**

FRESH COMMON THYME

## AND GUM INFECTIONS MOUTH/ULCERS

Bergamot, cinnamon leaf, cypress, sweet fennel, lemon, mastic, myrrh, orange (bitter and sweet), sage (clary and Spanish), thyme.
*Suggested application:* **S C**

## PSORIASIS

Angelica, bergamot, white birch, carrot seed, chamomile (German and Roman), true lavender.
*Suggested application:* **M S F B**

FRESH BERGAMOT

## RASHES

Peru balsam, Tolu balsam, carrot seed, chamomile (German and Roman), hops, true lavender, marigold, sandalwood, spikenard, tea tree, yarrow. *Suggested application:* **M S C F B**

## RINGWORM

Geranium, spike lavender, mastic, mint (peppermint and spearmint), myrrh, Levant styrax, tea tree, turpentine.
*Suggested application:* **S H**

FRESH SPEARMINT

## SCABIES

Tolu balsam, bergamot, cinnamon leaf, lavandin, lavender (spike and true), lemongrass, mastic, mint (peppermint and spearmint), Scotch pine, rosemary, Levant styrax, thyme, turpentine.
*Suggested application:* **S**

TRUE LAVENDER
LEAVES

## SCARS AND STRETCH MARKS

Cabreuva, elemi, frankincense, galbanum, true lavender, mandarin, orange blossom, palmarosa, patchouli, rosewood, sandalwood, spikenard, violet, yarrow.
*Suggested application:* **M S**

## SLACK TISSUE

Geranium, grapefruit, juniper, lemongrass, lime, mandarin, sweet marjoram, orange blossom, black pepper, petitgrain, rosemary, yarrow.
*Suggested application:* **M S B**

## SPOTS AND BLEMISHES

Bergamot, cade, cajeput, camphor (white), lemon-eucalyptus, helichrysum, lavandin, lavender (spike and true), lemon, lime, litsea cubeba, mandarin, niaouli, tea tree.
*Suggested application:*
**S N**

FRESH MANDARIN
LEAVES

## TICKS

Sweet marjoram.
*Suggested application:* **S N**

SWEET MARJORAM

## TOOTHACHE AND TEETHING PAIN

Chamomile (German and Roman), clove bud, mastic, mint (peppermint and spearmint), myrrh.
*Suggested application:* **S C N**

## VARICOSE VEINS

Cypress, lemon, lime, orange blossom, yarrow.
*Suggested application:* **S C**

## VERRUCAE
## (PLANTAR WARTS)

Tagetes, tea tree.
*Suggested application:* **S N**

LEAVES AND PEEL OF LIME

## WARTS AND CORNS

Cinnamon leaf, lemon, lime, tagetes, tea tree.
*Suggested application:* **S N**

## WOUNDS

Canadian balsam, Peru balsam, Tolu balsam, bergamot, cabreuva, chamomile (German and Roman), clove bud, cypress, elemi, eucalyptus (blue gum and lemon-scented), frankincense, galbanum, geranium, helichrysum, hyssop, juniper, lavandin, lavender (spike and true), linaloe, marigold, mastic, myrrh, niaouli, patchouli, rosewood, Levant styrax, tea tree, turpentine, vetiver, yarrow.
*Suggested application:* **S C B**

## WRINKLES AND MATURE SKIN

Carrot seed, elemi, sweet fennel, frankincense, galbanum, geranium, jasmine, labdanum, true lavender, mandarin, mimosa, myrrh, orange blossom, palmarosa, patchouli, rose (cabbage and damask), rosewood, clary sage, sandalwood, spikenard, ylang ylang.
*Suggested application:* **M S F B**

# Circulation, Muscles, and Joints

## ACCUMULATION OF TOXINS

Angelica, white birch, carrot seed, celery seed, cilantro, cumin, sweet fennel, grapefruit, juniper, lovage, parsley.
*Suggested application:* **M S B**

FRESH CILANTRO

## ACHES AND PAINS

Ambrette, star anise, aniseed, French basil, West Indian bay, cajeput, calamintha, camphor (white), chamomile (German and Roman), cilantro, eucalyptus (blue gum and peppermint), silver fir, galbanum, ginger, helichrysum, lavandin, lavender (spike and true), lemongrass, sweet marjoram, mastic, mint (peppermint and spearmint), niaouli, nutmeg, black pepper, pine (longleaf and Scotch), rosemary, sage (clary and Spanish), hemlock spruce, thyme, turmeric, turpentine, vetiver.
*Suggested application:* **M C B**

BLACK PEPPER

## ARTHRITIS

Allspice, angelica, benzoin, white birch, cajeput, camphor (white), carrot seed, cedarwood (Atlas, Texas, and Virginian), celery seed, chamomile (German and Roman), clove buds, cilantro, eucalyptus (blue gum and peppermint), silver fir, ginger, guaiacwood, juniper, lemon, sweet marjoram, mastic, myrrh, nutmeg, parsley, black pepper, pine (longleaf and Scotch), rosemary, Spanish sage, thyme, turmeric, turpentine, vetiver, yarrow.
*Suggested application:* **M S C B**

FRESH TURPENTINE

## CELLULITIS

White birch, cypress, sweet fennel, geranium, grapefruit, juniper, lemon, parsley, rosemary, thyme.
*Suggested application:* **M S B**

FRESH JUNIPER

## DEBILITY/POOR MUSCLE TONE

Allspice, ambrette, borneol, ginger, grapefruit, sweet marjoram, black pepper, pine (longleaf and Scotch), rosemary, Spanish sage.
*Suggested application:* **M S B**

AMBRETTE SEEDS

## EDEMA AND WATER RETENTION

Angelica, white birch, carrot seed, cypress, sweet fennel, geranium, grapefruit, juniper, lovage, mandarin, orange (bitter and sweet), rosemary, Spanish sage.
*Suggested application:* **M B**

## GOUT

Angelica, French basil, benzoin, carrot seed, celery seed, cilantro, guaiacwood, juniper, lovage, mastic, pine (longleaf and Scotch), rosemary, thyme, turpentine.
*Suggested application:* **M S B**

FRESH LOVAGE

## HIGH BLOOD PRESSURE AND HYPERTENSION

Lemon balm, cananga, garlic, true lavender, lemon, sweet marjoram, clary sage, yarrow, ylang ylang.
*Suggested application:* **M B V**

FRESH LEMON BALM

## MUSCULAR CRAMP AND STIFFNESS

Allspice, ambrette, cilantro, cypress, grapefruit, jasmine, lavandin, lavender (spike and true), sweet marjoram, black pepper, pine (longleaf and Scotch), rosemary, thyme, vetiver.
*Suggested application:*
**M C B**

FRESH JASMINE

## OBESITY

White birch, sweet fennel, juniper, lemon, mandarin, orange (bitter and sweet).
*Suggested application:*
**M B**

LEAVES AND PEEL OF SWEET ORANGE

## PALPITATIONS

Orange (bitter and sweet), orange blossom, rose (cabbage and damask), ylang ylang.
*Suggested application:* **M**

DRIED ROSE BUDS AND PETALS

## POOR CIRCULATION AND LOW BLOOD PRESSURE

Ambrette, Peru balsam, West Indian bay, benzoin, white birch, borneol, cinnamon leaf, cilantro, cumin, cypress, blue gum eucalyptus, galbanum, geranium, ginger, lemon, lemongrass, lovage, niaouli, nutmeg, orange blossom, black pepper, pine (longleaf and Scotch), rose (cabbage and damask), rosemary, Spanish sage, hemlock spruce, thyme, violet.
*Suggested application:* **M B**

FRESH HEMLOCK SPRUCE

## RHEUMATISM

Allspice, angelica, star anise, aniseed, Peru balsam, French basil, West Indian bay, benzoin, white birch, borneol, cajeput, calamintha, camphor (white), carrot seed, cedarwood (Atlas, Texas, and Virginian), celery seed, chamomile (German and Roman), cinnamon leaf, clove bud, cilantro, cypress, eucalyptus (blue gum and peppermint), sweet fennel, silver fir, galbanum, ginger, helichrysum, juniper, lavandin, lavender (spike and true), lemon, lovage, sweet marjoram, mastic, niaouli, nutmeg, parsley, black pepper, pine (longleaf and Scotch), rosemary, Spanish sage, hemlock spruce, thyme, turmeric, turpentine, vetiver, violet, yarrow. *Suggested application:* **M C B**

FRESH PERU BALSAM

## SPRAINS AND STRAINS

West Indian bay, borneol, camphor (white), chamomile (German and Roman), clove bud, eucalyptus (blue gum and peppermint), ginger, helichrysum, jasmine, lavandin, lavender (spike and true), sweet marjoram, black pepper, pine (longleaf and Scotch), rosemary, thyme, turmeric, vetiver. *Suggested application:* **C**

# Respiratory System

## ASTHMA

Asafetida, lemon balm, Canadian balsam, Peru balsam, benzoin, cajeput, clove bud, costus, cypress, elecampane, eucalyptus (blue gum, lemon-scented, and peppermint), frankincense, galbanum, helichrysum, hops, hyssop, lavandin, lavender (spike and true), lemon, lime, sweet marjoram, mint (peppermint and spearmint), myrrh, myrtle, niaouli, pine (longleaf and Scotch), rose (cabbage and damask), rosemary, sage (clary and Spanish), hemlock spruce, tea tree, thyme.
*Suggested application:* **M V I**

SWEET MARJORAM

## BRONCHITIS

Angelica, star anise, aniseed, asafetida, lemon balm, Canadian balsam, copaiba balsam, Peru balsam, Tolu balsam, French basil, benzoin, borneol, cajeput, camphor (white), caraway, cascarilla bark, cedarwood (Atlas, Texas, and Virginian), clove bud, costus, cubeb, cypress, elecampane, elemi, eucalyptus (blue gum and peppermint),silver fir, frankincense, galbanum, helichrysum, hyssop, labdanum, lavandin, lavender(spike and true), lemon, sweet marjoram, mastic, mint (peppermint and spearmint), myrrh, myrtle, niaouli, orange (bitter and sweet), pine (longleaf and Scotch), rosemary, sandalwood, hemlock spruce, Levant styrax, tea tree, thyme, turpentine, violet.
*Suggested application:* **M V I**

DRIED STAR ANISE

## CATARRH

Canadian balsam, Tolu balsam, cajeput, cedarwood (Atlas, Texas, and Virginian), cubeb, elecampane, elemi, eucalyptus (blue gum and peppermint), frankincense, galbanum, ginger, hyssop, jasmine, lavandin, lavender (spike and true), lemon, lime, mastic, mint (peppermint and spearmint), myrrh, myrtle, niaouli, black pepper, pine (longleaf and Scotch), sandalwood, Levant sytrax, tea tree, thyme, turpentine, violet.
*Suggested application:* **M V I**

FRESH ELECAMPANE

## CHILL

Copaiba balsam, benzoin, cabreuva, calamintha, camphor (white), cinnamon leaf, ginger, grapefruit, orange (bitter and sweet), black pepper.
*Suggested application:* **M B**

FRESH CALAMINTHA

## CHRONIC COUGHS

Lemon balm, Canadian balsam, costus, cubeb, cypress, elecampane, elemi, frankincense, galbanum, helichrysum, hops, hyssop, jasmine, mint (peppermint and spearmint), myrrh, myrtle, sandalwood, Levant styrax.
*Suggested application:*
**M V I**

FRESH GALBANUM FLOWERS

## COUGHS

Angelica, star anise, aniseed, copaiba balsam, Peru balsam, Tolu balsam, French basil, benzoin, borneol, cabreuva, cajeput, camphor (white), caraway, cascarilla bark, Atlas cedarwood, eucalyptus (blue gum and peppermint), silver fir, ginger, hyssop, labdanum, sweet marjoram, myrrh, niaouli, black pepper, pine (longleaf and Scotch), rose (cabbage and damask), rosemary, sage (clary and Spanish), hemlock spruce, tea tree.
*Suggested application:* **M V I**

LEVANT STYRAX

## CROUP

Tolu balsam.
*Suggested application:* **M I**

## EARACHE

French basil,
chamomile
(German and
Roman), lavender
(spike and true).
*Suggested
application:* **C**

TOLU
BALSAM

## HALITOSIS/OFFENSIVE BREATH

Bergamot, cardomon, sweet fennel, lavandin, lavender (spike
and true), mint (peppermint and spearmint), myrrh.
*Suggested application:* **S**

FRESH PEPPERMINT

## LARYNGITIS/HOARSENESS

Tolu balsam, benzoin, caraway, cubeb, lemon-scented
eucalyptus, frankincense, jasmine, lavandin, lavender
(spike and true), myrrh, sage (clary and Spanish),
sandalwood, thyme.
*Suggested
application:* **I**

FRESH SPANISH SAGE

## SINUSITIS

French basil, cajeput, cubeb, blue
gum eucalyptus, silver fir, ginger,
labdanum, peppermint, niaouli,
pine (longleaf and Scotch), tea tree.
*Suggested application:* **I**

ROOT OF GINGER

## SORE THROAT AND
## THROAT INFECTIONS

Canadian balsam, bergamot, cajeput, eucalyptus (blue gum,
lemon-scented and peppermint), geranium, ginger, hyssop,
lavandin, lavender (spike and true), myrrh, myrtle, niaouli,
pine (longleaf and Scotch), sage (clary and Spanish),
sandalwood, tea tree, thyme, violet.
*Suggested application:* **V I**

SCOTCH PINE

## TONSILLITIS

Bay laurel, bergamot, geranium, hyssop, myrtle, sage (clary
and Spanish), thyme. *Suggested application:* **I**

FRESH
COMMON THYME

## WHOOPING COUGH

Asafetida, helichrysum, hyssop, true lavender, mastic, niaouli,
rosemary, sage (clary and Spanish), tea tree, turpentine.
*Suggested application:* **M I**

TRUE LAVENDER

# Digestive System

## COLIC

Star anise, aniseed, lemon balm, calamintha, caraway, cardomon, carrot seed, chamomile (German and Roman), clove bud, cilantro, cumin, dill, sweet fennel, ginger, hyssop, lavandin, lavender (spike and true), sweet marjoram, mint (peppermint and spearmint), orange blossom, parsley, black pepper, rosemary, clary sage.
*Suggested application:* **M**

SPIKE LAVENDER

## CONSTIPATION AND SLUGGISH DIGESTION

Cinnamon leaf, cubeb, sweet fennel, lovage, sweet marjoram, nutmeg, orange (bitter and sweet), palmarosa, black pepper, tarragon, turmeric, yarrow.
*Suggested application:* **M B**

FRESH TARRAGON

## CRAMP/GASTRIC SPASM

Allspice, star anise, aniseed, caraway, cardomon, cinnamon leaf, cilantro, costus, cumin, galbanum, ginger, lavandin, lavender (spike and true), lovage, mint (peppermint and spearmint), orange blossom, black pepper, clary sage, tarragon, lemon verbena, yarrow.*Suggested application:* **M C**

FRESH YARROW

## GRIPING PAINS

Cardomon, dill, sweet fennel, parsley.
*Suggested application:* **M**

## HEARTBURN

Cardomon, black pepper. *Suggested application:* **M**

BLACK PEPPER

## INDIGESTION/FLATULENCE

Allspice, angelica, star anise, aniseed, lemon balm, French basil, bay laurel, calamintha, caraway, cardomon, carrot seed, cascarilla bark, celery seed, chamomile (German and Roman), cinnamon leaf, clove bud, cilantro, costus, cubeb, cumin, dill, sweet fennel, galbanum, ginger, hops, hyssop, lavandin, lavender (spike and true), lemongrass, linden, litsea cubeba, lovage, mandarin, sweet marjoram, mint (peppermint and spearmint), myrrh, nutmeg, orange (bitter and sweet), orange blossom, parsley, black pepper, petitgrain, rosemary, clary sage, tarragon, thyme, valerian, lemon verbena, yarrow.
*Suggested application:* **M**

FRESH LITSEA CUBEBA

## LIVER CONGESTION

Carrot seed, celery seed, helichrysum, linden, rose (cabbage and damask), rosemary, Spanish sage, turmeric, lemon verbena.
*Suggested application:* **M**

FRESH LEMON VERBENA

## LOSS OF APPETITE

Bay laurel, bergamot, caraway, cardomon, ginger, myrrh, black pepper.
*Suggested application:* **M**

## NAUSEA/VOMITING

Allspice, lemon balm, French basil, cardomon, cascarilla bark, chamomile (German and Roman), clove bud, cilantro, sweet fennel, ginger, lavandin, lavender (spike and true), mint (peppermint and spearmint), nutmeg, black pepper, rose (cabbage and damask), rosewood, sandalwood.
*Suggested application:*
**M V**

FRESH PARSLEY

FRESH ALLSPICE

# Genitourinary/Endocrine Systems

## AMENORRHEA/LACK OF MENSTRUATION

French basil, bay laurel, carrot seed, celery seed, cinnamon leaf, dill, sweet fennel, hops, hyssop, juniper, lovage, sweet marjoram, myrrh, parsley, rose (cabbage and damask), sage (clary and Spanish), tarragon, yarrow.

*Suggested application:* **M B**

FRESH DILL

## CYSTITIS

Canadian balsam, copaiba balsam, bergamot, cedarwood (Atlas, Texas, and Virginian), celery seed, chamomile (German and Roman), cubeb, blue gum eucalyptus, frankincense, juniper, lavandin, lavender (spike and true), lovage, mastic, niaouli, parsley, Scotch pine, sandalwood, tea tree, thyme, turpentine, yarrow.

*Suggested application:* **C B D**

## DYSMENORRHEA/CRAMP, PAINFUL OR DIFFICULT MENSTRUATION

Lemon balm, French basil, carrot seed, chamomile (German and Roman), cypress, frankincense, hops, jasmine, juniper, lavandin, lavender (spike and true), lovage, sweet marjoram, rose (cabbage and damask), rosemary, sage (clary and Spanish), tarragon, yarrow.

*Suggested application:* **M C B**

## FRIGIDITY

Cassie, cinnamon leaf, jasmine, nutmeg, orange blossom, parsley, patchouli, black pepper, cabbage rose, rosewood, clary sage, sandalwood, ylang ylang.

*Suggested application:* **M S B V**

## LABOR PAIN AND CHILDBIRTH AID

Cinnamon leaf, jasmine, true lavender, nutmeg, parsley, rose (cabbage and damask), clary sage.

*Suggested application:* **M C B**

## LACK OF NURSING MILK

Celery seed, dill, sweet fennel, hops.

*Suggested application:* **M**

## LEUCORRHEA/WHITE DISCHARGE FROM THE VAGINA

Bergamot, cedarwood (Atlas, Texas, and Virginian), cinnamon leaf, cubeb, blue gum eucalyptus, frankincense, hyssop, lavandin, lavender (spike and true), sweet marjoram, mastic, myrrh, rosemary, clary sage, sandalwood, tea tree, turpentine.

*Suggested application:* **B D**

## MENOPAUSAL PROBLEMS

Cypress, sweet fennel, geranium, jasmine, rose (cabbage and damask).

*Suggested application:* **M B V**

FRESH CYPRESS

## MENORRHAGIA/EXCESSIVE MENSTRUATION

Chamomile (German and Roman), cypress, rose (cabbage and damask).

*Suggested application:* **M B**

## PREMENSTRUAL SYNDROME/PMS

Carrot seed, chamomile (German and Roman), geranium, true lavender, sweet marjoram, orange blossom, tarragon.

*Suggested application:* **M B V**

## PRURITIS/ITCHING

Bergamot, Atlas cedarwood, juniper, lavender, myrrh, tea tree.

*Suggested application:* **D**

FRESH JUNIPER

## SEXUAL OVERACTIVITY

Hops, sweet marjoram.

*Suggested application:* **M B**

## THRUSH/CANDIDA

Bergamot, geranium, myrrh, tea tree.

*Suggested application:* **B D**

## URETHRITIS

Bergamot, cubeb, mastic, tea tree, turpentine.

*Suggested application:* **B D**

# Immune System

### CHICKENPOX

Bergamot, chamomile (German
and Roman), eucalyptus (blue
gum and lemon-scented), true
lavender, tea tree.

FRESH BERGAMOT

*Suggested application:* **C S B**

### COLDS/FLU

Angelica, star anise, aniseed, copaiba balsam, Peru balsam,
French basil, bay laurel, West Indian bay, bergamot, borneol,
cabreuva, cajeput, camphor (white), caraway, cinnamon leaf,
citronella, clove bud, cilantro, eucalyptus (blue gum, lemon-
scented, and peppermint), silver fir, frankincense, ginger,
grapefruit, helichrysum, juniper, lemon, lime, sweet marjoram,
mastic, mint (peppermint and spearmint), myrtle, niaouli,
orange (bitter and sweet), pine (longleaf and Scotch),
rosemary, rosewood,
Spanish sage, hemlock
spruce, tea tree, thyme,
turpentine, yarrow.
*Suggested application:*
**M B V I**

HEMLOCK SPRUCE

### FEVER

French basil, bergamot, borneol, camphor (white), eucalyptus
(blue gum, lemon-scented, and peppermint), silver fir, ginger,
helichrysum, juniper, lemon, lemongrass, lime, mint
(peppermint and spearmint), myrtle, niaouli, rosemary,
rosewood,
Spanish sage,
hemlock
spruce, tea tree,
thyme, yarrow.

FRESH NIAOULI

*Suggested application:* **C B**

### MEASLES

Bergamot, blue gum eucalyptus, lavender (spike and true),
tea tree.
*Suggested application:* **S B I V**

# Nervous System

### ANXIETY

Ambrette, lemon balm, French basil,
bergamot, cananga, frankincense, hyssop,
jasmine, juniper, true lavender, mimosa,
orange blossom, hemlock
spruce, Levant styrax, lemon
verbena, ylang ylang.
*Suggested application:*
**M B V**

LEVANT STYRAX

### DEPRESSION

Allspice, ambrette, lemon balm, Canadian balsam, French
basil, bergamot, cassie, grapefruit, helichrysum,
jasmine, true lavender, orange blossom, rose
(cabbage and damask), clary sage,
sandalwood, hemlock spruce,
vetiver, ylang ylang.

DRIED ROSE BUDS

*Suggested application:* **M B V**

### HEADACHE

Chamomile (German and Roman), citronella, cumin,
eucalyptus (blue gum and peppermint), grapefruit, hops,
lavandin, lavender (spike and true),
lemongrass, linden, sweet marjoram, mint
(peppermint and spearmint), rose
(cabbage and damask), rosemary,
rosewood, sage (clary and Spanish),
thyme, violet.
*Suggested application:* **M C V**

FRESH VIOLET

### INSOMNIA

Lemon balm, French basil, calamintha, chamomile (German
and Roman), hops, true lavender, linden, mandarin, sweet
marjoram, orange blossom, petitgrain, rose (cabbage and
damask), sandalwood, thyme, valerian, lemon verbena,
vetiver, violet, yarrow, ylang ylang.
*Suggested application:* **M B V**

## MIGRAINE

Angelica, lemon balm, French basil, chamomile (German and Roman), citronella, cilantro, true lavender, linden, sweet marjoram, mint (peppermint and spearmint), clary sage, valerian, yarrow. *Suggested application:* **C**

FRESH TRUE
LAVENDER

## NERVOUS EXHAUSTION OR FATIGUE/DEBILITY

Allspice, angelica, asafetida, French basil, borneol, cardomon, cassie, cinnamon leaf, citronella, cilantro, costus, cumin, elemi, eucalyptus (blue gum and peppermint), ginger, grapefruit, helichrysum, hyacinth, hyssop, jasmine, lavandin, spike lavender, lemongrass, mint (peppermint and spearmint), nutmeg, palmarosa, patchouli, petitgrain, Scotch pine, rosemary, sage (clary and Spanish), thyme, vetiver, violet, ylang ylang.
*Suggested application:* **M B V**

FRESH
HELICHRYSUM

## NERVOUS TENSION AND STRESS

Allspice, ambrette, angelica, asafetida, lemon balm, Canadian balsam, copaiba balsam, Peru balsam, French basil, benzoin, bergamot, borneol, calamintha, cananga, cardomon, cassie, cedarwood (Atlas, Texas, and Virginian), chamomile (German and Roman), cinnamon leaf, costus, cypress, elemi, frankincense, galbanum, geranium, helichrysum, hops, hyacinth, hyssop, jasmine, juniper, true lavender, lemongrass, linaloe, linden, mandarin, sweet marjoram, mimosa, mint

(peppermint and spearmint), orange (bitter and sweet), orange blossom, palmarosa, patchouli, petitgrain, Scotch pine, rose (cabbage and damask), rosemary, rosewood, clary sage, sandalwood, hemlock spruce, thyme, valerian, lemon verbena, vetiver, violet, yarrow, ylang ylang.
*Suggested application:* **M B V**

FRESH LINDEN

## NEURALGIA/SCIATICA

Allspice, West Indian bay, borneol, celery seed, chamomile (German and Roman), citronella, cilantro, eucalyptus (blue gum and peppermint), geranium, helichrysum, hops, spike lavender, sweet marjoram, mastic, mint (peppermint and spearmint), nutmeg, pine (longleaf and Scotch), rosemary, turpentine.
*Suggested application:* **M B**

FRESH SPEARMINT

## SHOCK

Lemon balm, lavandin, lavender (spike and true), orange blossom.
*Suggested application:* **M B V**

FRESH ORANGE

## VERTIGO

Lemon balm, lavandin, lavender (spike and true), mint (peppermint and spearmint), violet. *Suggested application:* **V I**

# The Oils

THE FOLLOWING PAGES *are a systematic survey of 167 essential oils, shown in alphabetical order according to the Latin name of the plants from which they are derived. The oils covered on these pages are all produced commercially, although some are little known or in scarce supply. A number of the oils have been designated as unsuitable for therapeutic use but have been included in this section for two reasons: first, to present a comprehensive picture of all the essential oils that are readily available; and second, to inform the reader about the possible dangers of such oils.*

*Aromatic plants are found all over the world, and essential oil production is an international industry, of which the "aromatherapy market" plays a small but rapidly expanding part. Individual entries contain a general description of the plant (illustrated in each case), the most up-to-date information about the actions of each essential oil, the methods of extraction, compatibilities with other oils (where relevant), a detailed guide to home and commercial uses, and safety data.*

BLENDED
OIL

SPEARMINT

BERGAMOT
SPRIG

LEFT *Frankincense is extracted from a small tree that is native to the Red Sea region and grows wild throughout northeast Africa. It has been used as an incense since ancient times in both Asia and the West.*

GRAPEFRUIT
LEAF

CHAMOMILE SPRIG

ORANGE
BLOSSOM LEAF

*ABELMOSCHUS MOSCHATUS*

# Ambrette seed

FAMILY: MALVACEAE

### Herbal/Folk Tradition

Generally used as a stimulant and to ease indigestion, cramp, and nervous dyspepsia. Widely used as a domestic spice in the East. In China it is used to treat headaches; in Egypt the seeds are used to sweeten the breath.

SEEDS

*An evergreen shrub about 5ft (1.5m) high, bearing large single yellow flowers with purple centers. The capsules, in the form of five-cornered pyramids, contain grayish-brown, kidney-shaped seeds that have a musky odor.*

## DATAFILE

**AROMATHERAPY/ HOME USE**
Circulation, Muscles, and Joints: *Cramp, fatigue, muscular aches and pains, poor circulation.*
Nervous System: *Anxiety, depression, nervous tension, and stress-related conditions.*

**EXTRACTION**
Essential oil by steam distillation of the seeds. Liquid ambrette seed should be allowed to age for several months before it is used. A concrete and absolute are also produced by solvent extraction.

**ACTIONS**
Antispasmodic, aphrodisiac, carminative, nervine, stimulant, stomachic.

**COMPATIBILITIES**
It blends well with rose, orange blossom, sandalwood, clary sage, cypress, patchouli, oriental, and "sophisticated" bases.

**SAFETY DATA**
*Nontoxic, nonirritant, and nonsensitizing*

---

*ABIES ALBA*

# Silver fir needle

FAMILY: PINACEAE

### Herbal/Folk Tradition

It is highly esteemed in Europe for its medicinal virtues and its fragrant scent. It is used mainly for respiratory complaints, fever, muscular and rheumatic pain.

SILVER FIR CONE

*A relatively small coniferous tree, with a regular pyramidal shape and a silvery white bark, grown chiefly for lumber and as Christmas trees.*

## DATAFILE

**AROMATHERAPY/ HOME USE**
Circulation, Muscles, and Joints: *Arthritis, muscular aches and pains, rheumatism.*
Respiratory System: *Bronchitis, coughs, sinusitis, etc.*
Immune System: *Colds, fever, flu.*

**EXTRACTION**
Essential oil by steam distillation from needles and young twigs, and from broken-up fir cones,

**ACTIONS**
Analgesic, antiseptic (pulmonary), antitussive, deodorant, expectorant, rubefacient, stimulant, tonic.

*Abies alba*

**COMPATIBILITIES**
It blends well with galbanum, labdanum, lavender, rosemary, lemon, pine, and marjoram.

**SAFETY DATA**
*Nontoxic, nonirritant (except in high concentration), nonsensitizing*

*ABIES BALSAMEA*

# Canadian balsam

FAMILY: PINACEAE

## Herbal/Folk Tradition

The oleoresin is used extensively by Native Americans for ritual purposes and as an external treatment for burns, sores, cuts, and to relieve heart and chest pains. It is also used internally for coughs.

DRIED CANADIAN BALSAM

*An evergreen tree up to 65ft (20m) high, with a tapering trunk and numerous branches, creating the overall shape of a perfect cone. It forms blisters of oleoresin (the so-called balsam) on the trunk and branches.*

### DATAFILE

**AROMATHERAPY/ HOME USE**

**Skin Care:** *Burns, cuts, hemorrhoids, wounds.*
**Respiratory System:** *Asthma, bronchitis, catarrh, chronic coughs, sore throat.*
**Genitourinary System:** *Cystitis, genitourinary infections.*
**Nervous System:** *Depression, nervous tension, stress-related conditions.*

**EXTRACTION**

The oleoresin is collected by puncturing vesicles in the bark. An essential oil is produced by steam distillation from the oleoresin (Canada balsam or Canada turpentine). Fir needle oil is produced by steam distillation from the leaf or needles.

**ACTIONS**

Antiseptic (genitourinary, pulmonary), antitussive, astringent, cicatrizant, diuretic, expectorant, purgative, regulatory, sedative (nerve), tonic, vulnerary.

**COMPATIBILITIES**

It blends well with pine, cypress, sandalwood, juniper, benzoin, and other balsams.

**SAFETY DATA**
*Generally nontoxic, nonirritant, nonsensitizing*

---

*ACACIA DEALBATA*

# Mimosa

FAMILY: MIMOSACEAE

## Herbal/Folk Tradition

The bark of mimosa ("wattle bark") has a leatherlike odor and astringent taste. It contains up to 42 per cent tannins (also gallic acid) and is used as a specific for diarrhea, and as an astringent gargle and ointment.

FRESH MIMOSA

*An attractive small tree up to 39ft (12m) high, having a grayish-brown bark with irregular, longitudinal ridges, delicate foliage, and clusters of fragrant yellow flowers.*

### DATAFILE

**AROMATHERAPY/ HOME USE**

**Skin Care:** *Oily, sensitive, general skin care.*
**Nervous System:** *Anxiety, nervous tension, oversensitivity, stress.*

**EXTRACTION**

A concrete and absolute by solvent extraction from the flowers and twig ends,

**ACTIONS**

Antiseptic, astringent.

**COMPATIBILITIES**

It blends well with lavandin, lavender, ylang, ylang, violet, styrax, cironella, Peru balsam,

*Acacia dealbata*

cassie, floral and spice oils. It is employed largely in soaps and also in high-quality perfumes, especially colognes, floral and oriental types.

**SAFETY DATA**
*Nontoxic, nonirritant, nonsensitizing*

*ACACIA FARNESIANA*

# Cassie

FAMILY: MIMOSACEAE

### Herbal/Folk Tradition

In India "attar of cassie" is made as a perfume. The fresh flowers are used in baths for dry skin. In Venezuela the root is used to treat stomach cancer. In China it is used to treat rheumatoid arthritis and pulmonary tuberculosis.

DRIED FLOWERS

*A bushy, thorny shrub, much branched, up to 33ft (10m) high. It has a very delicate appearance, similar to mimosa, with fragrant fluffy yellow flowers.*

### DATAFILE

**AROMATHERAPY/ HOME USE**
Use with care for:
Skin Care: *Dry, sensitive skin, perfume.*
Nervous System: *Depression, frigidity, nervous exhaustion, and stress-related conditions.*

**EXTRACTION**
An absolute by solvent extraction from the flowers.

**ACTIONS**
Antirheumatic, antiseptic, antispasmodic, aphrodisiac, balsamic, insecticide.

*Acacia farnesiana*

**COMPATIBILITIES**
It blends well with bergamot, costus, mimosa, frankincense, ylang ylang, orris, and violet and is used in high-quality perfumes, especially oriental types.

**SAFETY DATA**
*No available data on toxicity*

---

*ACHILLEA MILLEFOLIUM*

# Yarrow

FAMILY: ASTERACEAE (COMPOSITAE)

### Herbal/Folk Tradition

An age-old herbal medicine used for a wide variety of complaints including fever, respiratory infections, digestive problems, nervous tension, and externally for sores, rashes, and wounds.

FRESH YARROW

*A perennial herb with a simple stem up to 3ft (1m) high, with finely dissected leaves giving a lacy appearance, bearing numerous pinky-white, dense flowerheads.*

### DATAFILE

**AROMATHERAPY/ HOME USE**
Skin Care: *Acne, burns, cuts, eczema, hair rinse (promotes hair growth), inflammations, rashes, scars, varicose veins, wounds.*
Circulation, Muscles, and Joints: *Arteriosclerosis, high blood pressure, rheumatoid arthritis, thrombosis.*
Digestive System: *Constipation, cramp, flatulence, hemorrhoids, indigestion.*
Genitourinary System: *Amenorrhea, dysmenorrhea, cystitis, and other infections.*
Immune System: *Colds, fever, flu.*
Nervous System: *Hypertension, insomnia, stress.*

**EXTRACTION**
Essential oil by steam distillation from the dried herb.

**ACTIONS**
Anti-inflammatory, antipyretic, antirheumatic, antiseptic, antispasmodic, astringent, carminative, cicatrisant, diaphoretic, digestive, expectorant, hemostatic, hypotensive, stomachic, tonic.

**COMPATIBILITIES**
It blends well with cedarwood, pine, chamomile, valerian, vetiver, and oakmoss.

**SAFETY DATA**
*Non-toxic, non-irritant, possible sensitization in some individuals*

ACORUS CALAMUS VAR. ANGUSTATUS

# Calamus

FAMILY: ARACEAE

### Herbal/Folk Tradition

FRESH CALAMUS

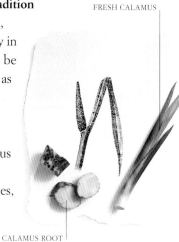

The aromatic oil, contained largely in the root, used to be highly esteemed as an aromatic stimulant and tonic for fever (typhoid), nervous complaints, vertigo, headaches, and dysentery.

CALAMUS ROOT

*A reedlike aquatic plant about 3ft (1m) high, with sword-shaped leaves and small greenish-yellow flowers. It grows on the margins of lakes and streams with the long-branched rhizome immersed in the mud.*

## DATAFILE

**AROMATHERAPY/ HOME USE**
None. "Should not be used in therapy, whether internally or externally."[2] It is extensively used in cosmetic and perfumery work, in woody/oriental/leather perfumes and to scent hair and tooth powders.

**EXTRACTION**
Essential oil by steam distillation from the rhizomes (and sometimes the leaves).

**ACTIONS**
Anticonvulsant, antiseptic, bactericidal, carminative, diaphoretic, expectorant,

*Acorus calamus var. angustatus*

hypotensive, insecticide, spasmolytic, stimulant, stomachic, tonic, vermifuge.

**COMPATIBILITIES**
It blends well with cananga, cinnamon, labdanum, olibanum, patchouli, cedarwood, amyris, spice and oriental bases.

### SAFETY DATA
*Oral toxin. The oil of calamus is reported to have carcinogenic properties*

---

AGOTHOSMA BETULINA

# Buchu

FAMILY: RUTACEAE

### Herbal/Folk Tradition

The leaves are used locally as an antiseptic and to ward off insects. In the West, the leaves are used for infections of the genitourinary system.

FRESH AND DRIED BUCHU

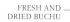

*A small, aromatic shrub with simple wrinkled leaves about ½in (1–2cm) long; other much smaller leaves are also present, which are bright green with finely serrated margins. Its delicate stems bear five-petaled white flowers.*

## DATAFILE

**AROMATHERAPY/ HOME USE**
None. A tincture, extract, and oleoresin are produced for pharmaceutical use. Limited use in blackcurrant flavor and fragrance work, for example, colognes and chypré bases.

**EXTRACTION**
Essential oil by steam distillation from the dried leaves.

**ACTIONS**
Antiseptic (especially urinary), carminative, diaphoretic, diuretic, insecticide, stimulant, tonic.

### SAFETY DATA
*Should not be used during pregnancy*

*ALLIUM CEPA*

# Onion

FAMILY: LILIACEAE

### Herbal/Folk Tradition

Onion has an ancient
reputation as a
curative agent. It is
high in vitamins A, B,
and C. Raw onion
helps to keep
infections and colds
at bay, promotes
strong bones, and a
good blood supply. It
is an effective blood
cleanser and keeps the
skin clear.

ONION SKIN

ONION SEED

*A perennial or biennial herb up to 4ft (1.2m) high
with hollow leaves and flowering stem, and a globelike,
fleshy bulb.*

### DATAFILE

**AROMATHERAPY/
HOME USE**
None, due to its offensive,
sulfuraceous smell. It is,
however, used in some
pharmaceutical preparations for
colds, coughs, etc. The oil is
used extensively in most major
food categories, especially
meats, savories, and salad
dressings.

**EXTRACTION**
Essential oil by steam distillation
from the bulb. (An oleoresin is
also produced in small
quantities for flavoring use).

**ACTIONS**
Anthelmintic, antimicrobial,
antirheumatic, antiseptic,
antisclerotic, antispasmodic,
antiviral, bactericidal,
carminative, depurative,
digestive, diuretic, expectorant,
fungicidal, hypocholesterolemic,
hypoglycemic, hypotensive,
stomachic, tonic, vermifuge.

**SAFETY DATA**
*Specific safety data unavailable at present – probably similar to garlic,
i.e. generally nontoxic, nonirritant, possible sensitization*

---

*ALLIUM SATIVUM*

# Garlic

FAMILY: AMARYLLIDACEAE OR LILIACEAE

### Herbal/Folk Tradition

Used for thousands of
years for respiratory
and urinary tract
infections, digestive
problems, heart
disease, high blood
pressure, epidemics
and fever.

GARLIC BULB

CLOVE OF GARLIC

*A strongly scented perennial herb up to 4ft (1.2m) high
with long, flat, firm leaves and whitish flowering stems.
The bulb is made up of several cloves pressed together
within a thin white skin.*

### DATAFILE

**AROMATHERAPY/
HOME USE**
Due to its unpleasant and
pervasive smell, the oil is not
often used externally. However,
the capsules may be taken
internally according to the
instructions on the label for
respiratory and gastrointestinal
infections, urinary tract
infections such as cystitis, heart
and circulatory problems, and
to fight infectious diseases in
general.

**EXTRACTION**
Essential oil by steam distillation
from the fresh crushed bulbs.

**ACTIONS**
Amoebicidal, anthelmintic,
antibiotic, antimicrobial,
antiseptic, antitoxic, antitumor,
antiviral, bactericidal,
carminative, cholagogue,
hypocholesterolemic,
depurative, diaphoretic, diuretic,
expectorant, febrifuge,
fungicidal, hypoglycemic,
hypotensive, insecticidal,
larvicidal, promotes
leucocytosis, stomachic, tonic.

**SAFETY DATA**
*Generally nontoxic and nonirritant, although it has been known to
irritate the stomach; may also cause sensitization in some individuals*

*ALOYSIA TRIPHYLLA*

# Lemon verbena

FAMILY: VERBENACEAE

## Herbal/Folk Tradition

Lemon verbena is indicated especially in nervous conditions that manifest as digestive complaints. The dried leaves are used as a tea, both as a refreshing "pick-me-up" and to help restore the liver after a hangover.

FRESH LEMON VERBENA

*A handsome deciduous perennial shrub up to 16ft (5m) high with a woody stem, very fragrant, delicate, pale green, lanceolate leaves arranged in threes, and small, pale purple flowers. Often grown as an ornamental bush.*

### DATAFILE

**AROMATHERAPY/ HOME USE**

**Digestive System:** *Cramps, indigestion, liver congestion.*
**Nervous System:** *Anxiety, insomnia, nervous tension, and stress-related conditions.*
True verbena oil is virtually non-existent. Most so-called verbena oil is either from the Spanish verbena
(an inferior oil) or a mix of lemongrass, lemon, citronella, etc.

**EXTRACTION**

Essential oil by steam distillation from the freshly harvested herb.

**ACTIONS**

Antiseptic, antispasmodic, carminative, detoxifying, digestive, febrifuge, hepatobiliary stimulant, sedative (nervous), stomachic.

**COMPATIBILITIES**

It blends well with neroli, palmarosa, olibanum, Tolu balsam, elemi, lemon, and other citrus oils.

**SAFETY DATA**
*Possible sensitization; phototoxicity due to high citral levels. Other saftey data is unavailable at present*

---

*ALPINIA OFFICINARUM*

# Galangal

FAMILY: ZINGIBERACEA

## Herbal/Folk Tradition

It is used as a local spice, especially in curries; in India it is employed in perfumery. The root is current in the British Herbal Pharmacopoeia, indicated for dyspepsia, flatulence, colic, nausea, and vomiting.

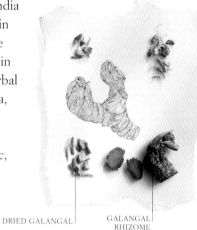

DRIED GALANGAL

GALANGAL RHIZOME

*A reedlike plant reaching a height of about 3ft (1m), with irregularly branched rhizomes red or brown on the outside, light orange within.*

### DATAFILE

**AROMATHERAPY/ HOME USE**

(Possibly digestive upsets.) It is also used as a flavor ingredient, especially in spice and meat products, and is occasionally used in perfumery.

**EXTRACTION**

Essential oil by steam distillation from the rhizomes. (An oleoresin is also produced by solvent extraction.)

**ACTIONS**

Antiseptic, bactericidal, carminative, diaphoretic, stimulant, stomachic.

**COMPATIBILITIES**

It blends well with chamomile maroc, sage, cinnamon, allspice, lavandin, pine needle, rosemary, patchouli, myrtle, opopanax, and citrus oils.

**SAFETY DATA**
*Safety data unavailable at present*

*AMYRIS BALSAMIFERA*

# Amyris

FAMILY: RUTACEAE

## Herbal/Folk Tradition

Locals call this bushy tree, which originated in Haiti and is cultivated in tropical zones all over the world, "candle wood" because of its high oil content; it burns like a candle. It is used as a torch by fishermen and traders. It also makes excellent furniture wood.

AMYRIS CHIPPINGS

*A small bushy tree with compound leaves and white flowers, which grows wild in thickets all over the island of Haiti.*

DATAFILE

**AROMATHERAPY/
HOME USE**
Perfume.

**EXTRACTION**
Essential oil by steam distillation from the broken-up wood and branches. Best if the wood is seasoned first. It provides a very plentiful yield.

**ACTIONS**
Antiseptic, balsamic, sedative.

**COMPATIBILITIES**
It blends well with lavandin, citronella, oakmoss, sassafras, cedarwood, and wood oils.

**SAFETY DATA**
*Nontoxic, nonirritant, nonsensitizing*

---

*ANETHUM GRAVEOLENS*

# Dill

FAMILY: APIACEAE (UMBELLIFERAE)

## Herbal/Folk Tradition

Used since the earliest times as a medicinal and culinary herb, especially in Germany and Scandinavia. In the West and East it is used as a digestive aid for indigestion, wind, colic, etc., especially in children.

FRESH DILL

*Annual or biennial herb up to 3ft (1m) high with a smooth stem, feathery leaves and umbels of yellowish flowers followed by flat, small seeds.*

DATAFILE

**AROMATHERAPY/
HOME USE**
Digestive System: *Colic, dyspepsia, flatulence, indigestion.*
Genitourinary and Endocrine Systems: *Lack of periods; promotes milk flow in nursing mothers.*

**EXTRACTION**
Essential oil by steam distillation from fruit or seed, and herb or weed (fresh or partially dried).

**ACTIONS**
Antispasmodic, bactericidal, carminative, digestive, emmenagogue, galactagogue, hypotensive, stimulant, stomachic.

*Anethum graveolens*

**COMPATIBILITIES**
It blends well with elemi, mint, caraway, nutmeg, and spice and citrus oils.

**SAFETY DATA**
*Nontoxic, nonirritant, nonsensitizing*

# Angelica

FAMILY: APIACEAE (UMBELLIFERAE)

## Herbal/Folk Tradition

This herb has been praised for its virtues since antiquity. It strengthens the heart, stimulates the circulation and the immune system. It is used for rheumatic inflammation, bronchial ailments, colds, indigestion, wind, and as an appetite stimulant and urinary antiseptic.

FRESH ANGELICA

SECTION OF
FRESH STALK

ANGELICA ROOT

*A large, hairy plant with ferny leaves and umbels of white flowers. It has a strong aromatic scent and a large rhizome.*

### DATAFILE

**AROMATHERAPY/ HOME USE**

**Skin Care:** *Dull congested skin, irritated conditions, psoriasis.*
**Circulation, Muscles, and Joints:** *Accumulation of toxins, arthritis, gout, rheumatism, water retention.*
**Respiratory System:** *Bronchitis, coughs.*
**Digestive System:** *Anemia, anorexia, flatulence, indigestion.*
**Nervous System:** *Fatigue, migraine, nervous tension, and stress-related disorders.*
**Immune System:** *Colds.*

**EXTRACTION**
Essential oil produced by steam distillation from the roots and rhizomes, and fruit or seed.

**ACTIONS**
Antispasmodic, carminative, depurative, diaphoretic, digestive, diuretic, emmenagogue, expectorant, febrifuge, nervine, stimulant, stomachic, tonic.

**COMPATIBILITIES**
It blends well with patchouli, opopanax, costus, clary sage, oakmoss, veitiver, and citrus oils.

**SAFETY DATA**
*Both root and seed oil are nontoxic and nonirritant. The root oil (not the seed oil) is phototoxic, probably due to higher levels of bergapten. Not to be used during pregnancy or by diabetics*

---

# Rosewood

FAMILY: LAURACEAE

## Herbal/Folk Tradition

Used for building, carving, and French cabinet-making. Nowadays, most rosewood goes to Japan for the production of chopsticks.

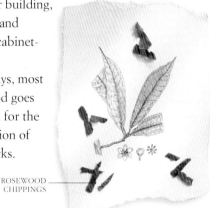

ROSEWOOD
CHIPPINGS

*Medium-size, tropical, evergreen tree with a reddish bark and heartwood, bearing yellow flowers. Used extensively for lumber. NB: Rosewood is being extensively felled in the clearing of the South American rainforests; the production of rosewood oil is consequently environmentally damaging.*

### DATAFILE

**AROMATHERAPY/ HOME USE**

**Skin Care:** *Acne, dermatitis, scars, wounds, wrinkles, and general skin care: sensitive, dry, dull, combination oily/dry, etc. "Although it does not have any dramatic curative power I find it very useful especially for skin care. It is very mild and safe to use."*[3]
**Immune System:** *Colds, coughs, fever, infections, stimulates the immune system.*
**Nervous System:** *Frigidity, headaches, nausea, nervous tension, and stress-related conditions.*

**EXTRACTION**
Essential oil by steam distillation of the wood chippings.

**ACTIONS**
Mildly analgesic, anticonvulsant, antidepressant, antimicrobial, antiseptic, aphrodisiac, bactericidal, cellular stimulant, cephalic, deodorant, stimulant (immune system), tissue regenerator, tonic.

**COMPATIBILITIES**
It blends well with most oils, especially citrus, woods, and florals. It helps give body and rounds off sharp edges.

**SAFETY DATA**
*Nontoxic, nonirritant, nonsensitizing*

## *ANTHRISCUS CEREFOLIUM*

# Chervil

FAMILY: APIACEAE (UMBELLIFERAE)

### Herbal/Folk Tradition

The leaves are used as a domestic spice. In folk medicine it is used as a tea to tone up the blood and nerves, and for poor memory and depression. Juice is used for skin ailments such as eczema, abscesses, and slow-healing wounds.

SPRIG OF FRESH CHERVIL

*An annual herb up to 12in (30cm) high, with a slender, much-branched stem, bright green, finely divided, fernlike leaves, umbels of flat white flowerheads and long smooth seeds or fruits. It has an aromatic scent when bruised.*

**DATAFILE**

**AROMATHERAPY/HOME USE**
None. Methyl chavicol and anethole are known to have toxic and irritant effects; methyl chavicol is reported to have possible carcinogenic effects. Since these constitute the major proportion of the essential oil, it is best avoided for therapeutic use.

**EXTRACTION**
Essential oil by steam distillation from seeds or fruit

**ACTIONS**
Aperitif, antiseptic, carminative, cicatrisant, depurative, diaphoretic, digestive, diuretic, nervine, restorative, stimulant (metabolism), stomachic, tonic.

*Anthriscus cerefolium*

**SAFETY DATA**
*Toxic and irritant effects; possibly carcinogenic effects*

## *APIUM GRAVEOLENS*

# Celery seed

FAMILY: APIACEAE (UMBELLIFERAE)

### Herbal/Folk Tradition

The seed is used in bladder and kidney complaints, digestive upsets, and menstrual problems; the leaves are used in skin ailments. It is known to increase the elimination of uric acid and is useful for gout, neuralgia, and rheumatoid arthritis.

CELERY SEED

*A familiar biennial plant, 12–24in (30–60cm) high, with a grooved, fleshy, erect stalk, shiny pinnate leaves, and umbels of white flowers.*

**DATAFILE**

**AROMATHERAPY/HOME USE**
Circulation, Muscles, and Joints: *Arthritis, buildup of toxins in the blood, gout, rheumatism.*
Digestive System: *Dyspepsia, flatulence, indigestion, liver congestion, jaundice.*
Genitourinary and Endocrine Systems: *Amenorrhea, glandular problems, increases milk flow, cystitis.*
Nervous System: *Neuralgia, sciatica.*

**EXTRACTION**
Essential oil by steam distillation from whole or crushed seeds. An oil from the whole herb; an oleoresin, and extract are also produced in small quantities.

**ACTIONS**
Antioxidative, antirheumatic, antiseptic (urinary), antispasmodic, aperitif, depurative, digestive, diuretic, carminative, cholagogue, emmenagogue, galactagogue, hepatic, nervine, sedative (nervous), stimulant (uterine), stomachic, tonic (digestive).

**COMPATIBILITIES**
It blends well with lavender, pine, opopanax, lovage, tea tree, oakmoss, cilantro, and other spices.

**SAFETY DATA**
*Nontoxic, nonirritant, possible sensitization. Avoid during pregnancy*

*ARMORACIA RUSTICANA*

# Horseradish

FAMILY: BRASSICACEAE (CRUCIFERAE)

### Herbal/Folk Tradition

An extremely stimulating herb, once valued as a household remedy. It was used for fever, digestive complaints, urinary infections, and as a circulatory aid. Good for arthritis and rheumatism.

HORSERADISH ROOT

SECTION OF ROOT

*A perennial plant with large leaves up to 20in (50cm) long, white flowers, and a thick, whitish, tapering root, which is propagated easily.*

## DATAFILE

### AROMATHERAPY/ HOME USE

None. This essential oil should not be used in therapy either externally or internally. It is used mainly in minute amounts in seasonings, ready-made salads, condiments, and canned products.

### EXTRACTION

Essential oil by water and steam distillation from the broken roots that have been soaked in water. (A resinoid or concrete is also produced by solvent extraction.)

*Armoracia rusticana*

### ACTIONS

Antibiotic, antiseptic, diuretic, carminative, expectorant, laxative (mild), rubefacient, stimulant.

### SAFETY DATA

Oral toxin, dermal irritant, mucous membrane irritant

---

*ARNICA MONTANA*

# Arnica

FAMILY: ASTERACEAE (COMPOSITAE)

### Herbal/Folk Tradition

This herb stimulates the peripheral blood supply when applied externally, and is one of the best remedies for bruises and sprains. It is never used internally.

DRIED ARNICA PETALS

*A perennial alpine herb with a creeping underground stem, giving rise to a rosette of pale oval leaves. The flowering, erect stem is up to 24in (60cm) high, bearing a single, bright yellow, daisylike flower. The plant is difficult to cultivate.*

## DATAFILE

### AROMATHERAPY/ HOME USE

None.

### EXTRACTION

Essential oil by steam distillation of flowers and root. The yield of essential oil is very small. An absolute, tincture, and resinoid are also produced.

### ACTIONS

Anti-inflammatory, stimulant, vulnerary.

*Arnica montana*
*Native to northern and central Europe, also found growing wild in Russia, Scandinavia, and northern India.*

### SAFETY DATA

The essential oil is highly toxic and should never be used internally or on broken skin. However, the tincture or arnica ointment are valuable additions to the home medicine cabinet

*ARTEMISIA ABSINTHIUM*

# Wormwood

FAMILY: ASTERACEAE (COMPOSITAE)

## Herbal/Folk Tradition

Used as an aromatic-bitter for anorexia, as a digestive tonic, and as a choleretic for liver and gall bladder disorders, usually in the form of a dilute extract. It is also used to promote menstruation, reduce fever, and expel worms.

FRESH WORMWOOD

*A perennial herb up to 5ft (1.5m) high with a whitish stem, silvery-green, divided leaves covered with silky, fine hairs, and pale yellow flowers.*

| DATAFILE |
| :---: |

**AROMATHERAPY/ HOME USE**
None. This oil should not be used in therapy. Habitual use can cause restlessness, nightmares, convulsions, vomiting, and, in extreme cases, brain damage. In 1915 the French banned the production of the drink absinthe with this plant, because of its narcotic and habit-forming properties.

**EXTRACTION**
Essential oil by steam distillation from the leaves and flowering tops. (An absolute is occasionally produced by solvent extraction.)

**ACTIONS**
Anthelmintic, choleretic, deodorant, emmenagogue, febrifuge, insect repellant, narcotic, stimulant (digestive), tonic, vermifuge.

**COMPATIBILITIES**
It blends well with oakmoss, jasmine, orange blossom, lavender, and hyacinth.

**SAFETY DATA**
*Toxic. Abortifacient*

---

*ARTEMISIA DRACUNCULUS*

# Tarragon

FAMILY: ASTERCEAE (COMPOSITAE)

## Herbal/Folk Tradition

The leaf is commonly used as a domestic herb and to make tarragon vinegar. The maharajahs of India took it as a tisane, and in Persia it was used to induce appetite. The leaf was also used for digestive and menstrual irregularities.

FRESH TARRAGON

*A perennial herb with smooth narrow leaves; an erect stem up to 1.2m (4ft) tall, and small yellowy-green, inconspicuous flowers.*

| DATAFILE |
| :---: |

**AROMATHERAPY/ HOME USE**
Digestive System: *Anorexia, dyspepsia, flatulence, hiccoughs, intestinal spasm, nervous indigestion, sluggish digestion.*
Genitourinary System: *Amenorrhea, dysmenorrhea, PMS.*

**EXTRACTION**
Essential oil by steam distillation from the leaves.

**ACTIONS**
Anthelmintic, antiseptic, antispasmodic, aperitif, carminative, digestive, diuretic, emmenagogue, hypnotic, stimulant, stomachic, vermifuge.

**COMPATIBILITIES**
It blends well with labdanum, galbanum, lavender, oakmoss, vanilla, pine, and basil.

**SAFETY DATA**
*Moderately toxic due to "estragole" (methyl chavicol): use in moderation only. Possibly carcinogenic. Otherwise nonirritant, nonsensitizing. Avoid during pregnancy*

*ARTEMISIA VULGARIS*

# Mugwort

FAMILY: ASTERACEAE (COMPOSITAE)

### Herbal/Folk Tradition

Associated, in Europe, with witchcraft and superstition. It was seen as a woman's plant, used as a womb tonic, for painful, delayed menstruation, and for hysteria and epilepsy. It was also used to expel worms, control fever, and as a digestive remedy.

DRIED MUGWORT LEAVES

*An erect, much-branched, perennial herb up to 5ft (1.5m) high, with purplish stems, dark green divided leaves that are downy white beneath, and numerous small reddish-brown or yellow flowers.*

## DATAFILE

**AROMATHERAPY/ HOME USE**
None. It should not be used in therapy either internally or externally. It is, however, used as a fragrance component in soaps, colognes, and perfumes.

**EXTRACTION**
Essential oil by steam distillation from the leaves and flowering tops.

**ACTIONS**
Anthelmintic, antispasmodic, carminative, choleretic, diaphoretic, diuretic, emmenagogue, nervine, orexigenic, stimulant, stomachic, tonic (uterine, womb), vermifuge.

**COMPATIBILITIES**
It blends well with oakmoss, patchouli, rosemary, lavandin, pine, sage, clary sage, and cedarwood.

**SAFETY DATA**
*Oral toxin, due to high thujone content. Abortifacient*

---

*ASARUM CANADENSE*

# Snakeroot

FAMILY: ARISTOLOCHIACEAE

### Herbal/Folk Tradition

This plant has been used for centuries in folk medicine but is now little prescribed. It was used for chronic chest complaints, rheumatism, dropsy, and painful bowel and stomach spasms.

FRESH SNAKEROOT

*A fragrant little plant not more than 14in (35cm) high with hairy stem, two glossy, kidney-shaped leaves, and a creeping rootstock. The solitary bell-shaped flower is brownish purple, and creamy white inside.*

## DATAFILE

**AROMATHERAPY/ HOME USE**
May possibly be used for its antispasmodic qualities, for example, for period pains or indigestion.

**EXTRACTION**
Essential oil by steam distillation from dried rhizomes and crushed roots.

**ACTIONS**
Anti-inflammatory, antispasmodic, carminative, diuretic, diaphoretic, emmenagogue, expectorant, febrifuge, stimulant, stomachic.

**COMPATIBILITIES**
It blends well with bergamot, costus, oakmoss, patchouli, pine needle, clary sage, mimosa, cassie, and other florals.

**SAFETY DATA**
*Nontoxic, nonirritant, nonsensitizing. Avoid during pregnancy*

*BETULA ALBA*

# White birch

FAMILY: BETULACEAE

## Herbal/Folk Tradition

Birch buds were formerly used as a tonic in hair preparations. Birch tar is used in Europe for chronic skin complaints, such as psoriasis, eczema. In Scandinavia the sap is tapped and drunk as a tonic, and birch leaflets and twigs are used in the sauna.

DRIED LEAVES

*Decorative tree, up to 49–65ft (15–20m) high, with slender branches, silvery-white bark broken into scales, and light green oval leaves. The male catkins are 1–2in (2–5cm) long, the female up to 6in (15cm) long.*

### DATAFILE

**AROMATHERAPY/ HOME USE**

**Skin Care:** *Dermatitis, dull or congested skin, eczema, hair care, psoriasis, etc.*

**Circulation, Muscles, and Joints:** *Accumulation of toxins, arthritis, cellulitis, muscular pain, obesity, edema, poor circulation, rheumatism.*

**EXTRACTION**

Essential oil by steam distillation from the leaf-buds. Crude birch tar is also extracted by slow destructive distillation from the bark; this is subsequently steam-distilled to yield a rectified birch tar oil.

**ACTIONS**

Anti-inflammatory, antiseptic, cholagogue, diaphoretic, diuretic, febrifuge, tonic.

**COMPATIBILITIES**

It blends well with other woody and balsamic oils.

**SAFETY DATA**
*Nontoxic, nonirritant, nonsensitizing*

---

*BETULA LENTA*

# Sweet birch

FAMILY: BETULACEAE

## Herbal/Folk Tradition

The cambium (the layer directly under the bark) is eaten in the spring. Bark infusion is used as a stimulant and to promote sweating. As a decoction or syrup, it is used as a tonic for dysentery.

AROMATIC BARK

A SPRIG OF SWEET BIRCH

*A graceful tree about 82ft (25m) high, which has a pyramidal shape while young. It has bright green leaves and a dark reddish-brown aromatic bark, which is broken into plates or patches.*

### DATAFILE

**AROMATHERAPY/ HOME USE**

None. Methyl salicylate can be absorbed through the skin, and can cause fatal poisoning. It is also classed as an environmental hazard or marine pollutant.

**EXTRACTION**

Essential oil by steam distillation of the bark macerated in water.

**ACTIONS**

Analgesic, anti-inflammatory, antipyretic, antirheumatic, antiseptic, astringent, depurative, diuretic, rubefacient, tonic.

*Betula lenta*
*Native to southern Canada and eastern United States. Produced mainly in Pennsylvania.*

**SAFETY DATA**
*Methyl salicylate, the major constituent, is not exactly toxic but very harmful in concentration*

## BORONIA MEGASTIGMA

# Boronia

FAMILY: RUTACEAE

### Herbal/Folk Tradition

A botanist in the Victorian era suggested this species would be suitable for graveyard planting because of its dark flowers!

DRIED FLOWERS

*A bushy evergreen shrub, up to 6ft (2m) high, which bears an abundance of fragrant, nodding flowers with an unusual coloring – the petals are brown on the outside, yellow on the inside. Often grown as an ornamental shrub in gardens.*

## DATAFILE

**AROMATHERAPY/ HOME USE**
Perfume.

**EXTRACTION**
A concrete and absolute by the enfleurage method or petroleum-ether extraction, from the flowers. Essential oil is by steam distillation.

**ACTIONS**
Aromatic.

**COMPATIBILITIES**
It blends well with clary sage, sandalwood, bergamot, violet, helichrysum, costus, mimosa, and other florals.

*Boronia megastigma
Native to Western Australia; grows wild all over west and southwest Australia.*

### SAFETY DATA
*Prohibitively expensive and therefore often adulterated*

---

## BRASSICA NIGRA

# Mustard

FAMILY: BRASSICACEAE (CRUCIFERAE)

### Herbal/Folk Tradition

The seeds are highly esteemed as a condiment and for their medicinal qualities. Used to aid digestion, and promote the appetite, and for colds, chills, coughs, chilblains, rheumatism, arthritis, lumbago, and aches and pains.

MUSTARD SEED

*An erect annual up to 10ft (3m) high, with spear-shaped upper leaves, smooth flat pods containing about ten dark brown seeds, and yellow flowers.*

## DATAFILE

**AROMATHERAPY/ HOME USE**
None. It is not recommended for therapy, either externally or internally.

**EXTRACTION**
Essential oil by steam (or water) distillation from the black mustard seeds, which have been macerated in warm water.

**ACTIONS**
Aperitif, antimicrobial, antiseptic, diuretic, emetic, febrifuge, rubefacient (produces blistering of the skin), stimulant.

*Brassica nigra
Common throughout eastern Europe, southern Siberia, Asia Minor, and North Africa; naturalized in North and South America.*

### SAFETY DATA
*Oral toxin, dermal toxin, mucous membrane irritant. It is considered one of the most toxic of all essential oils*

*BOSWELLIA CARTERI*

# Frankincense

FAMILY: BURSERACEA

## Herbal/Folk Tradition

Used since antiquity as an incense in India, China, and in the West by the Catholic Church. In ancient Egypt it was used in rejuvenating face masks, cosmetics, and perfumes. It has been used medicinally in the East and West for a wide range of conditions including syphilis, rheumatism, respiratory and urinary tract infections, skin diseases, as well as digestive and nervous complaints. In addition, frankincense is extensively used in the manufacture of incense, and the gum and oil are used as fragrance components in soaps, cosmetics, and perfumes, especially oriental fragrances.

*A pale yellow or greenish mobile liquid with a fresh, terpeney top note and a warm, rich, sweet-balsamic undertone. A handsome small tree or shrub with abundant pinnate leaves and white or pale pink flowers. It yields a natural oleo gum resin.*

GUM RESIN

---

**DATAFILE**

### AROMATHERAPY/ HOME USE

**Skin Care:** *Blemishes, dry and mature complexions, scars, wounds, wrinkles.*

**Respiratory System:** *Asthma, bronchitis, catarrh, coughs, laryngitis.*

**Genitourinary System:** *Cystitis, dysmenorrhea, leucorrhea, metrorrhagia.*

**Immune System:** *Colds, flu.*

**Nervous System:** *Anxiety, nervous tension, and stress: "Frankincense has, among its physical properties, the ability to slow down and deepen the breath … which is very conducive to prayer and meditation."*[4]

### EXTRACTION

Essential oil by steam distillation from oleo gum resin (approx. 3–10 per cent oil to 60–70 per cent resin). An absolute is also produced, used mainly as a fixative.

### ACTIONS

Anti-inflammatory, antiseptic, astringent, carminative, cicatrizant, cytophylactic, digestive, diuretic, emmenagogue, expectorant, sedative, tonic, uterine, vulnerary.

*Boswellia Carteri*

### COMPATIBILITIES

It blends well with sandalwood, pine, vetiver, geranium, lavender, mimosa, orange, bergamot, camphor, basil, pepper, and other spices.

---

**SAFETY DATA**
*Nontoxic, nonirritant, nonsensitizing*

# Calamintha

FAMILY: LAMIACEAE (LABIATAE)

## Herbal/Folk Tradition

It has a long history of use as a herbal remedy mainly for nervous and digestive complaints, also menstrual pain, colds, chills, and cramp. Catmint is current in the British Herbal Pharmacopoeia as a specific for flatulent colic in children and for the common cold. Catmint is native to Europe and parts of Asia, and naturalized throughout South Africa and North America, where it is used as a wild cat lure. It is cultivated for its oil throughout the Mediterranean region, former Yugoslavia, Poland and in the USA.

*An erect, bushy, perennial plant not more than 3ft (1m) high, with square stems, soft oval serrated leaves grayish-green beneath, and rather inconspicuous pale purple flowers. The whole plant has a strong aromatic scent, which is attractive to cats.*

FRESH LEAF

---

**DATAFILE**

### AROMATHERAPY/ HOME USE
**Circulation, Muscles, and Joints:**
*Chills, cold in the joints, muscular aches and pains, rheumatism.*
**Digestive System:**
*Colic, flatulence, nervous dyspepsia.*
**Nervous System:**
*Insomnia, nervous tension, and stress-related conditions.*

### EXTRACTION
Essential oil by steam distillation from the flowering tops.

### ACTIONS
Anesthetic (local), antirheumatic, antispasmodic, astringent, carminative, diaphoretic, emmenagogue, febrifuge, nervine, sedative, tonic.

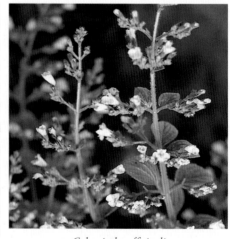

*Calamintha officinalis*

**SAFETY DATA**
*Nontoxic, nonirritant, nonsensitizing*

*BURSERA GLABRIFOLIA*

# Linaloe

FAMILY: BURSERACEAE

### Herbal/Folk Tradition

The seed oil is known in India as "Indian lavender oil" and used chiefly as a local perfume ingredient and in soaps by the cosmetics industry of Mysore state. It is not much found outside India.

LINALOE
CHIPPINGS

*A tall, bushy tropical shrub or tree, with a smooth bark and bearing fleshy fruit. The wood is used only for distillation purposes when the tree is twenty or thirty years old. The oil is stimulated by lacerating the trunk.*

### DATAFILE

**AROMATHERAPY/ HOME USE**
Skin Care: *Acne, cuts, dermatitis, wounds, etc., all skin types.*
Nervous System: *Nervous tension and stress-related conditions.*

**EXTRACTION**
Essential oil by steam distillation from the wood and seed and husk. (An essential oil is also occasionally produced from the leaves and twigs.)

**ACTIONS**
Anticonvulsant, anti-inflammatory, antiseptic, bactericidal, deodorant, gentle tonic.

**COMPATIBILITIES**
It blends well with rose, sandalwood, cedarwood, rosewood, frankincense, floral and woody fragrances.

### SAFETY DATA
*Nontoxic, nonirritant, nonsensitizing*

---

*BULNESIA SARMIENTI*

# Guaiacwood

FAMILY: ZYGOPHYLLACEAE

### Herbal/Folk Tradition

Guaiacwood was once used for treating rheumatism and gout, and is still current in the *British Herbal Pharmacopoeia* as a specific for rheumatism and rheumatoid arthritis.

GUAIACWOOD
SAWDUST

*A small, wild, tropical tree up to 13ft (4m) high.*

### DATAFILE

**AROMATHERAPY HOME USE**
Circulation, Muscles, and Joints: *Arthritis, gout, rheumatoid arthritis.*

**EXTRACTION**
Essential oil by steam distillation from the broken wood and sawdust. The fluid extract and tincture are used in pharmacology, mainly as a diagnostic reagent in blood texts. Used as a fixative and fragrance component in soaps, cosmetics, and perfumes. Guaiacwood oil is used as a flavor component in most categories of food product as well as in drinks.

**ACTIONS**
Anti-inflammatory, antioxidant, antirheumatic, antiseptic, diaphoretic, diuretic, laxative.

**COMPATIBILITIES**
It blends well with geranium, orange blossom, oakmoss, rose, costus, sandalwood, amyris, spice and woody-floral bases.

### SAFETY DATA
*Nonirritant, nonsensitizing; possible toxic effects in concentration. Use in moderation. Avoid during pregnancy*

*CALENDULA OFFICINALIS*

# Marigold

FAMILY: ASTERACEAE (COMPOSITAE)

## Herbal/Folk Tradition

A herb of ancient medical repute, used for skin complaints, menstrual irregularities, varicose veins, hemorrhoids, conjunctivitis, and poor eyesight. The infused oil is used for a wide range of skin problems.

MARIGOLD PETALS

FLOWER HEAD

*An annual herb up to 24in (60cm) high with soft, oval, pale green leaves and bright orange, daisylike flowers.*

### DATAFILE

**AROMATHERAPY/ HOME USE**

The infused oil is very valuable in aromatherapy for its powerful skin-healing properties.

**Skin Care:** *Burns, cuts, eczema, greasy skin, inflammations, insect bites, rashes, wounds.*

**EXTRACTION**

An absolute by solvent extraction from the flowers. The real calendula absolute is produced only in small quantities and is difficult to get hold of.

**ACTIONS**

Antihemorrhagic, anti-inflammatory, antiseptic, antispasmodic, astringent, diaphoretic, cholagogue, cicatrizant, emmenagogue, febrifuge, fungicidal, styptic, tonic, vulnerary.

**COMPATIBILITIES**

It blends well with oakmoss, hyacinth, floral, and citrus oils.

**SAFETY DATA**

*Nontoxic, nonirritant, nonsensitizing*

---

*CANANGA ODORATA VAR. GENUINA*

# Ylang ylang

FAMILY: ANNONACEAE

## Herbal/Folk Tradition

In the Molucca Islands, an ointment is made from ylang ylang and cucuma flowers for cosmetic and hair care, skin diseases, to prevent fever and fight infections.

DRIED YLANG YLANG BARK

*A tall tropical tree up to 65ft (20m) high with large, tender, fragrant flowers, which can be pink, mauve, or yellow.*

### DATAFILE

**AROMATHERAPY/ HOME USE**

**Skin Care:** *Acne, hair growth, hair rinse, insect bites, irritated and oily skin, general skin care.*

**Circulation, Muscles, and Joints:** *High blood pressure, hypernea, tachycardia, palpitations.*

**Nervous System:** *Depression, frigidity, impotence, insomnia, nervous tension, and stress. "…soothes and inhibits anger."[5]*

**EXTRACTION**

Essential oil by water or steam distillation from the freshly picked flowers. The first distillation (about 40 per cent)

is called ylang ylang extra, which is the top grade. An absolute and concrete are also produced by solvent extraction.

**ACTIONS**

Aphrodisiac, antidepressant, anti-infectious, antiseborrheic, antiseptic, euphoric, hypotensive, nervine, regulator, sedative, stimulant, tonic.

**COMPATIBILITIES**

It blends well with rosewood, jasmine, vetiver, opopanax, bergamot, mimosa, cassie, Peru balsam, rose, tuberose, and costus,

**SAFETY DATA**

*Nontoxic, nonirritant, possible sensitization especially in those with sensitive skin*

*CANANGA ODORATA*

# Cananga

FAMILY: ANNONACEAE

### Herbal/Folk Tradition

Used locally for infectious illnesses, for example, malaria. The beautiful flowers are also used for decorative purposes at festivals. Cananga is very closely related to the tree that produces ylang ylang oil, but is considered an inferior product in perfumery work; being grown in different regions, the oil has a different quality, being heavier and less delicate than ylang ylang. However, cananga is truly a "complete" oil, whereas ylang ylang is made into several distillates.

*Cananga oil is a greenish-yellow or orange viscous liquid with a sweet, floral-balsamic tenacious scent.*

*A tall tropical tree, up to 98ft (30m) high, which flowers all year round. It bears large, fragrant, tender, yellow flowers that are virtually identical to those of the ylang ylang.*

FRESH LEAF

---

## DATAFILE

### AROMATHERAPY/ HOME USE
**Skin Care:** *Insect bites, fragrance, general skin care.*
**Nervous Systems:** *Anxiety, depression, nervous tension, and stress-related complaints.*

### EXTRACTION
Essential oil by water distillation from the flowers

### ACTIONS
Antiseptic, antidepressant, aphrodisiac, hypotensive, nervine, sedative, tonic.

### COMPATIBILITIES
It blends well with calamus, birch tar, copaiba balsam, labdanum, orange blossom, oakmoss, jasmine, guaiacwood, and oriental-type bases.

*Cananga odorata*

---

### SAFETY DATA
*Nontoxic, nonirritant, a few cases of sensitization reported. Use in moderation, since its heady scent can cause headaches or nausea*

*CANARIUM LUZONICUM*

# Elemi

FAMILY: BURSERACEAE

## Herbal/Folk Tradition

The gum or oleoresin is used locally for skin care, respiratory complaints, and as a general stimulant. Elemi was one of the aromatics used by the ancient Egyptians for the embalming process.

ELEMI RESIN

*A tropical tree up to 98ft (30m) high that yields a resinous pathological exudation with a pungent odor. Although it is called a gum, it is almost entirely made up of resin and essential oil.*

### DATAFILE

**AROMATHERAPY/ HOME USE**
Skin Care: *Aged skin, infected cuts and wounds, inflammations, rejuvenation, wrinkles – "signifies drying and preservation."[6]*
Respiratory System: *Bronchitis, catarrhal conditions, dry coughs.*
Nervous System: *Nervous exhaustion and stress-related conditions.*

**EXTRACTION**
Essential oil by steam distillation from the gum. (A resinoid and resin absolute are also produced in small quantities.)

**ACTIONS**
Antiseptic, balsamic, cicatrizant, expectorant, fortifying, regulatory, stimulant, stomachic, tonic.

**COMPATIBILITIES**
It blends well with myrrh, frankincense, labdanum, rosemary, lavender, lavandin, sage, cinnamon, and other spices.

**SAFETY DATA**
*Nontoxic, nonirritant, nonsensitizing*

---

*CARPHEPHORUS ODORATISSIMUS*

# Deertongue

FAMILY: ASTERACEAE (COMPOSITAE)

## Herbal/Folk Tradition

The roots have been used for their diuretic effects, and applied locally for sore throats and gonorrhea. It is a tonic, used to treat malaria. In folklore it is associated with contraception and sterility in women.

DRIED DEERTONGUE LEAVES

*A herbaceous perennial plant distinguished by a naked receptacle and feathery pappus, with large, fleshy, dark green leaves, clasped at the base. The dried leaves have a vanilla-like odor.*

### DATAFILE

**AROMATHERAPY/ HOME USE**
None.

**EXTRACTION**
Oleoresin by solvent extraction from the dried leaves.

**ACTIONS**
Antiseptic, demulcent, diaphoretic, diuretic, febrifuge, stimulant, tonic.

**COMPATIBILITIES**
It blends well with oakmoss, labdanum, lavandin, frankincense, clove, patchouli, and oriental-type fragrances.

**SAFETY DATA**
*"Coumarin has toxic properties including liver injury and hemorrhages."[7] Possible dermal irritation and phototoxicity due to the lactones present*

*CARUM CARVI*

# Caraway

FAMILY: APIACEAE (UMBELLIFERAE)

### Herbal/Folk Tradition

Used extensively as a domestic spice. Traditional remedy for dyspepsia, intestinal colic, menstrual cramps, poor appetite, laryngitis and bronchitis. It promotes milk secretion and is considered specific for flatulent colic in children.

CURVED CARAWAY SEEDS

*A biennial herb up to 2½ft (75cm) high with a much-branched stem, finely cut leaves, and umbels of white flowers, with a thick and tapering root.*

## DATAFILE

### AROMATHERAPY/ HOME USE

**Respiratory System:** *Bronchitis, coughs, laryngitis.*
**Digestive System:** *Dyspepsia, colic, flatulence, gastric spasm, nervous indigestion, poor appetite. See also sweet fennel and dill.*
**Immune System:** *Colds.*

### EXTRACTION

Essential oil by steam distillation from the dried ripe seed or fruit (approximate 2–8 per cent yield).

### ACTIONS

Antihistaminic, antimicrobial, antiseptic, aperitif, astringent, carminative, diuretic, emmenagogue, expectorant, galactagogue, larvicidal, stimulant, spasmolytic, stomachic, tonic, vermifuge.

### COMPATIBILITIES

It blends well with jasmine, cinnamon, cassia and other spices; however, it is very overpowering.

### SAFETY DATA

*Nontoxic, nonsensitizing; may cause dermal irritation in concentration*

---

*CEDRUS ATLANTICA*

# Atlas cedarwood

FAMILY: PINACEAE

### Herbal/Folk Tradition

The oil from the Lebanon cedar was used by the ancient Egyptians for embalming, cosmetics, and perfumery. Traditionally used in the East for bronchial and urinary tract infections, as a preservative, and as an incense.

ATLAS CEDARWOOD CONE

*Pyramid-shaped majestic evergreen tree, up to 131ft (40m) high. The wood itself is hard and strongly aromatic because of the high percentage of essential oil it contains.*

## DATAFILE

### AROMATHERAPY/ HOME USE

**Skin Care:** *Acne, dandruff, dermatitis, eczema, fungal infections, greasy skin, hair loss, skin eruptions, ulcers.*
**Circulation, Muscles, and Joints:** *Arthritis, rheumatism.*
**Respiratory System:** *Bronchitis, catarrh, congestion, coughs.*
**Genitourinary System:** *Cystitis, leucorrhea, pruritis.*
**Nervous System:** *Nervous tension and stress-related conditions.*

### EXTRACTION

Resinoid, absolute, and essential oil by steam distillation from wood, stumps, and sawdust.

### ACTIONS

Antiseptic, antiputrescent, antiseborrheic, aphrodisiac, astringent, diuretic, expectorant, fungicidal, mucolytic, sedative (nervous), stimulant (circulatory), tonic.

### COMPATIBILITIES

It blends well with rosewood, bergamot, boronia, cypress, calamus, cassie, costus, jasmine, juniper, neroli, mimosa, labdanum, olibanum, clary sage, vetiver, rosemary, ylang ylang, oriental and flower bases.

### SAFETY DATA

*Nontoxic, nonirritant, nonsensitizing. Best avoided during pregnancy*

*CHAMAEMELUM NOBILE*

# Roman chamomile

FAMILY: ASTERACEAE (COMPOSITAE)

## Herbal/Folk Tradition

This herb has had a medical reputation in Europe and especially in the Mediterranean region for over 2,000 years, and it is still in widespread use. It was employed by the ancient Egyptians and the Moors, and it was one of the Saxons' nine sacred herbs, which they called "maythen". It was also held to be the "plant's physician", since it promoted the health of plants nearby.

It is current in the *British Herbal Pharmacopoeia* for the treatment of dyspepsia, nausea, anorexia, vomiting in pregnancy, dysmenorrhea, and specifically flatulent dyspepsia associated with mental stress.

*A small, stocky, perennial herb, up to 25cm (10in) high, with a much-branched hairy stem, half spreading or creeping. It has feathery pinnate leaves and daisylike white flowers.*

DRIED ROMAN CHAMOMILE

FRESH PINNATE LEAVES

---

### DATAFILE

### AROMATHERAPY/ HOME USE

**Skin Care:** *Acne, allergies, boils, burns, cuts, chilblains, dermatitis, earache, eczema, hair care, inflammations, insect bites, rashes, sensitive skin, teething pain, toothache, wounds.*

**Circulation, Muscles, and Joints:** *Arthritis, inflamed joints, muscular pain, neuralgia, rheumatism, sprains.*

**Digestive System:** *Dyspepsia, colic, indigestion, nausea.*

**Genitourinary System:** *Dysmenorrhea, menopausal problems, menorrhagia.*

**Nervous System:** *Headache, insomnia, nervous tension,*

*migraine, and stress-related complaints.*

### EXTRACTION

Essential oil by steam distillation of the flowerheads. Used in antiseptic ointments and in carminative, antispasmodic, and tonic preparations. Extensively used in cosmetic, soaps, detergents, high-quality perfumes, and hair and bath products.

### ACTIONS

Analgesic, antianemic, antineuralgic, antiphlogistic, antiseptic, antispasmodic, bactericidal, carminative,

*Citrus nobile*

cholagogue, cicatrizant, digestive, emmenagogue, febrifuge, hepatic, hypnotic, nerve sedative, stomachic, sudorific, tonic, vermifuge, vulnerary.

### COMPATIBILITIES

It blends well with bergamot, clary sage, oakmoss, jasmine, labdanum, orange blossom, rose, geranium, and lavender.

---

### SAFETY DATA

*Nontoxic, nonirritant; can cause dermatitis in some individuals*

*CHENOPODIUM AMBROSIOIDES VAR. ANTHELMINTICUM*

# Wormseed

FAMILY: CHENOPODIACEAE

### Herbal/Folk Tradition

Several Native American tribes of the eastern United States use the whole of the herb decocted to help ease painful menstruation and other female complaints. It is also used to expel roundworm, hookworm, and dwarf tapeworm.

DRIED FLOWERS

*A hairy, coarse, perennial wayside herb up to 3ft (1m) high with stout, erect stem, oblong-lanceolate leaves, and many greenish-yellow flowers, the same color as the leaves.*

## DATAFILE

### AROMATHERAPY/ HOME USE

None. "It should not be used in therapy, either internally or externally, and is one of the most toxic essential oils."[8] Cases of fatal poisoning have been reported even in low doses. Effects can be cumulative. Due to high ascaridole content, the oil may explode when heated or treated with acids.

### EXTRACTION

Essential oil by steam distillation from the whole herb, especially fruit or seeds.

*Chenopodium ambrosioides var. anthelminticum Native to South America; cultivated mainly in east and southeast United States, also India, Hungary, and Russia.*

### ACTIONS

Anthelmintic, antirheumatic, antispasmodic, expectorant, hypotensive.

### SAFETY DATA

A very toxic oil

---

*CINNAMOMUM CAMPHORA*

# Camphor

FAMILY: LAURACEAE

### Herbal/Folk Tradition

A long-standing traditional protection against infectious disease. In addition it was used for nervous and respiratory diseases in general, and for heart failure. It is very poisonous in large doses.

CAMPHOR BARK

*A tall, handsome, evergreen tree, up to 98ft (30m) high. It has many branches bearing clusters of small white flowers followed by red berries. The wood of mature trees produces a white crystalline substance, the crude camphor.*

## DATAFILE

### AROMATHERAPY/ HOME USE

Brown and yellow camphor should not be used in therapy. White camphor may be used with care for:

**Skin Care:** *Acne, blemishes, inflammation, oily conditions; also for insect prevention.*

**Circulation, Muscles, and Joints:** *Arthritis, muscular aches and pains, rheumatism, sprains, etc.*

**Respiratory System:** *Bronchitis, chills, coughs.*

**Immune System:** *Colds, fever, flu, infectious diseases.*

### EXTRACTION

Crude camphor oil is collected from trees in crystalline form. The essential oil is produced by steam distillation from the wood, root stumps, and branches and then rectified under vacuum and filter pressed to produce three fractions, known as white, brown, and yellow camphor.

### ACTIONS

Anti-inflammatory, antiseptic, antiviral, bactericidal, counter-irritant, diuretic, expectorant, stimulant, rubefacient, vermifuge.

### SAFETY DATA

Brown and yellow camphor (containing safrol) are toxic and carcinogenic. White camphor does not contain safrol and is relatively nontoxic, nonsensitizing, and nonirritant. Not compatible with homeopathic treatment

# Cassia

FAMILY: LAURACEAE

## Herbal/Folk Tradition

Extensively used as a local domestic spice. It is used medicinally mainly for digestive complaints such as flatulent dyspepsia, colic, diarrhea, and nausea, as well as the common cold, rheumatism, and kidney and reproductive complaints.

DRIED CASSIA STALKS

*A slender, evergreen tree up to 65ft (20m) high, with leathery leaves and small white flowers. The fruit is approximately the size of a small olive.*

### DATAFILE

**AROMATHERAPY/ HOME USE**
None. It should never be used on the skin and is one of the most hazardous oils.

**EXTRACTION**
Essential oil by steam distillation from the leaves, and by water distillation from the bark, leaves, twigs, and stalks.

**ACTIONS**
Antidiarrheal, antiemetic, antimicrobial, astringent, carminative, spasmolytic.

**SAFETY DATA**
*Dermal toxin, dermal irritant, dermal sensitizer, mucous membrane irritant*

---

# Labdanum

FAMILY: CISTACEAE

## Herbal/Folk Tradition

One of the early aromatic substances of the ancient world. The gum was used for catarrh, diarrhea, dysentery, and to promote menstruation; externally it was used in plasters.

LANCE-SHAPED LEAVES

FRESH FLOWER

*A small sticky shrub up to 10ft (3m) high with lance-shaped leaves that are white and furry on the underside, and fragrant white flowers. Labdanum gum is a natural oleoresin, obtained by boiling the plant material in water.*

### DATAFILE

**AROMATHERAPY/ HOME USE**
Skin Care: *Mature skin, wrinkles.*
Respiratory System: *Coughs, bronchitis, rhinitis, etc.*
Immune System: *Colds.*

**EXTRACTION**
A resinoid or resin concrete and absolute by solvent extraction from the crude gum. An essential oil by steam distillation from the crude gum, the absolute, or from the leaves and twigs of the plant.

**ACTIONS**
Antimicrobial, antiseptic, antitussive, astringent, balsamic, emmenagogue, expectorant, tonic.

**COMPATIBILITIES**
It blends well with oakmoss, clary sage, pine, juniper, calamus, opopanax, lavender, lavandin, bergamot, cypress, veitiver, sandalwood, patcholi, olibanum, and maroc chamomile.

**SAFETY DATA**
*Generally nontoxic, nonirritant, nonsensitizing. Avoid during pregnancy*

*CINNAMOMUM ZEYLANICUM*

# Cinnamon

FAMILY: LAURACEAE

## Herbal/Folk Tradition

The inner bark of the new shoots from the cinnamon tree are gathered every two years and used in the form of sticks as a domestic spice. It has been used for thousands of years in the East for a variety of complaints, including colds, flu, digestive and menstrual problems, rheumatism, kidney troubles, and as a general stimulant. Current in the British Herbal Pharmacopoeia as a specific for flatulent colic and dyspepsia with nausea.

*A yellow to brownish liquid with a warm, spicy, somewhat harsh odor.*

*A tropical evergreen up to 49ft (15m) high, with strong branches and thick scabrous bark with young shoots speckled greeny-orange. It has shiny green leaves, small white flowers, and oval berries.*

CRUSHED CINNAMON

STICKS OF CINNAMON

---

**DATAFILE**

### AROMATHERAPY/ HOME USE
Cinnamon bark oil – none. It is one of the most hazardous oils, and should never be used on the skin.
Cinnamon leaf oil:
Skin Care: *Lice, scabies, tooth and gum care, warts, wasp stings.*
Circulation, Muscles, and Joints: *Poor circulation, rheumatism.*
Digestive System: *Anorexia, colitis, diarrhea, dyspepsia, intestinal infection, sluggish digestion, spasm.*
Genitourinary System: *Childbirth (stimulates contractions), frigidity, leucorrhea,* *metrorrhagia, scanty periods.*
Immune System: *Chills, colds, flu, infectious diseases.*
Nervous System: *Debility, nervous exhaustion, and stress-related conditions.*

### EXTRACTION
Essential oil by water or steam distillation from the leaves and twigs, and from the dried inner bark.

### ACTIONS
Anthelmintic, antidiarrheal, antidote (to poison), antimicrobial, antiseptic, antispasmodic, antiputrescent, aphrodisiac, astringent, carminative, digestive, emmenagogue, hemostatic, orexigenic, parasiticide, refrigerant, spasmolytic, stimulant (circulatory, cardiac, respiratory), stomachic, vermifuge.

### COMPATIBILITIES
It blends well with olibanum, ylang ylang, orange mandarin, benzoin, and Peru balsam.

*Cinnamon zeylanicum*

---

**SAFETY DATA**
*1. Leaf oil is relatively nontoxic; possibly irritant because of the cinnamaldehyde. Eugenol is irritant to the mucous membranes: use in moderation. 2. Bark oil is a dermal toxin, irritant, and sensitizer; also irritant to the mucous membranes*

*CITRUS AURANTIFOLIA*

# Lime

FAMILY: RUTACEAE

## Herbal/Folk Tradition

The fruit is often used indiscriminately in place of lemon with which it shares many qualities. It is used for similar purposes including fever, infections, sore throat, colds, etc. In the past was used as a remedy for dyspepsia with glycerin of pepsin.

FRUIT PEEL

*A small evergreen tree up to 15ft (4.5m) high, with stiff sharp spines, smooth ovate leaves, and small white flowers. The bitter fruit is pale green, about half the size of a lemon.*

### DATAFILE

**AROMATHERAPY/ HOME USE**

**Skin Care:** *Acne, anemia, blemishes, brittle nails, boils, chilblains, corns, cuts, greasy skin, herpes, insect bites, mouth ulcers, varicose veins, warts.*

**Circulation, Muscles, and Joints:** *Arthritis, cellulitis, high blood pressure, nosebleeds, obesity (congestion), poor circulation, rheumatism.*

**Respiratory System:** *Asthma, throat infections, bronchitis, catarrh.*

**Digestive System:** *Dyspepsia.*

**Immune System:** *Colds, flu, fever and infections.*

**EXTRACTION**

Essential oil by cold expression of the peel of the unripe fruit (preferred in perfumery work) or by steam distillation of the whole ripe crushed fruit (a by-product of the juice industry).

**ACTIONS**

Antirheumatic, antiscorbutic, antiseptic, antiviral, aperitif, bactericidal, febrifuge, restorative, tonic.

**COMPATIBILITIES**

It blends well with neroli, citronella, lavender, lavandin, rosemary, clary sage, and other citrus oils.

**SAFETY DATA**

*Nontoxic, nonirritant, nonsensitizing. However, the expressed "peel" oil is phototoxic (but not the steam-distilled "whole fruit" oil)*

---

*CITRUS AURANTIUM VAR. AMARA*

# Bitter orange

FAMILY: RUTACEAE

## Herbal/Folk Tradition

The dried bitter orange peel is used as a tonic and carminative in treating dyspepsia. Ingestion of large amounts of orange peel in children, however, is said to cause toxic effects.

FLOWER PETALS

OUTER PEEL OF FRUIT

FRESH BITTER ORANGE

*An evergreen tree up to 33ft (10m) high with dark green, glossy, oval leaves, with long spines. It has a smooth grayish trunk and branches, and fragrant white flowers. The fruits are smaller and darker than the sweet orange.*

### DATAFILE

**AROMATHERAPY/ HOME USE**

See Sweet Orange page 72.

**EXTRACTION**

An essential oil by cold expression (hand or machine pressing) from the outer peel of the almost ripe fruit. (A terpeneless oil is also produced.) The leaves are used for the production of petitgrain oil; the blossom for neroli oil.

**ACTIONS**

Anti-inflammatory, antiseptic, astringent, bactericidal,

*Citrus aurantium var. amara*

carminative, choleretic, fungicidal, sedative (mild), stomachic, tonic.

**SAFETY DATA**

*Phototoxic; otherwise generally nontoxic, nonirritant and nonsensitizing. Limonene has been reported to cause contact dermatitis in some individuals*

*CITRUS AURANTIUM VAR. AMARA*

# Orange blossom

FAMILY: RUTACEAE

FLOWER PETAL

### Herbal/Folk Tradition

This oil, neroli, was named after a princess of Nerola in Italy, who wore it as a perfume. Orange flowers have many folk associations. They were used in bridal bouquets: to calm nervous apprehension before the couple retired to the marriage bed.

In Europe an infusion of dried flowers is used as a mild stimulant of the nervous system, and as a blood cleanser. The distillation water, known as orange flower water, is a popular cosmetic and household article.

*The essential oil is a dark yellow or brownish yellow mobile liquid with a fresh, dry almost floral odor.*

*An evergreen tree up to 33ft (10m) high with glossy dark green leaves and fragrant white flowers.*

ORANGE BLOSSOM LEAVES

---

**DATAFILE**

### AROMATHERAPY/ HOME USE

**Skin Care:** *Scars, stretch marks, thread veins, mature and sensitive skin, tones the complexion, wrinkles.*

**Circulation, Muscles, and Joints:** *Palpitations, poor circulation.*

**Digestive system:** *Diarrhea (chronic), colic, flatulence, spasm, nervous dyspepsia.*

**Nervous system:** *Anxiety, depression, nervous tension, PMS, shock, stress-related conditions – "I find that by far the most important uses of neroli are in helping with problems of emotional origin."*[9]

### EXTRACTION

A concrete and aboslute are produced by solvent extraction from the freshly picked flowers, and an essential oil is produced by steam distillation. An orange flower water and an absolute are produced as a by-product of the distillation process.

### ACTIONS

Antidepressant, antiseptic, antispasmodic, aphrodisiac, bactericidal, carminative, cicatrizant, cordial, deodorant, digestive, fungicidal, hypnotic (mild), stimulant (nervous), tonic (cardiac, circulatory).

*Citrus sinensis*

### COMPATIBILITIES

It blends well with virtually all oils: chamomile, coriander, geranium, benzoin, clary sage, jasmine, lavender, rose, ylang ylang, lemon, and other citrus oils.

---

**SAFETY DATA**
*Nontoxic, nonirritant, nonsensitizing, nonphototoxic*

*CITRUS AURANTIUM VAR. AMARA*

# Petitgrain
FAMILY: RUTACEAE

## Herbal/Folk Tradition
At one time the oil used to be extracted from the green unripe oranges when they were still the size of cherries – hence the name petitgrains or "little grains". One of the classic ingredients of eau-de-cologne.

FRESH PETITGRAIN

*The oil of petitgrain is produced from the leaves and twigs of the same tree that produces bitter orange oil and orange blossom oil: see Bitter orange, page 68 and Orange blossom, page 69.*

### DATAFILE

**AROMATHERAPY/ HOME USE**

**Skin Care:** *Acne, excessive perspiration, greasy skin and hair, toning.*

**Digestive System:** *Dyspepsia, flatulence.*

**Nervous System:** *Convalescence, insomnia, nervous exhaustion, and stress-related conditions.*

**EXTRACTION**
Essential oil by steam distillation from the leaves and twigs. An orange "leaf and flower" water absolute is also produced, known as *petitgrain sur fleurs.*

**ACTIONS**
Antiseptic, antispasmodic, deodorant, digestive, nervine, stimulant (digestive, nervous), stomachic, tonic.

**COMPATIBILITIES**
It blends well with rosemary, lavender, geranium, bergamot, bitter orange, orange blossom, labdanum, oakmoss, clary sage, jasmine, benzoin, palmarosa, clove, and balsams.

### SAFETY DATA
*Nontoxic, nonirritant, nonsensitizing, nonphototoxic*

---

*CITRUS BERGAMIA*

# Bergamot
FAMILY: RUTACEAE

## Herbal/Folk Tradition
Named after the city of Bergamot in Lombardy, where the oil was first sold. The oil has been used in Italy for many years, primarily for worms and fever (including malaria). Also useful for mouth, skin, respiratory, and urinary tract infections.

FRESH BERGAMOT

*A small tree, about 15ft (4.5m) high with smooth oval leaves, bearing small round fruit that ripen from green to yellow, much like a miniature orange in appearance.*

### DATAFILE

**AROMATHERAPY/ HOME USE**

**Skin Care:** *Acne, blemishes, boils, cold sores, eczema, insect repellent and bites, oily skin, psoriasis, scabies, varicose ulcers, wounds.*

**Respiratory System:** *Halitosis, mouth infections, sore throat.*

**Digestive System:** *Flatulence, loss of appetite.*

**Genitourinary System:** *Cystitis, leucorrhea, pruritis, thrush.*

**Immune System:** *Colds, fever, flu, infectious diseases.*

**Nervous System:** *Anxiety, depression, and stress.*

**EXTRACTION**
Essential oil by cold expression of the peel of the fruit.

**ACTIONS**
Analgesic, anthelmintic, antidepressant, antiseptic (pulmonary, genitourinary), antispasmodic, antitoxic, carminative, digestive, diuretic, deodorant, febrifuge, laxative, parasiticide, rubefacient, stimulant, stomachic, tonic, vermifuge, vulnerary.

### SAFETY DATA
*Certain furocoumarins, notably bergapten, have been found to be phototoxic in concentration and in dilution even after some time. Extreme care must be taken in dermal applications – or substitute with a rectified or "bergapten-free" oil. Otherwise nontoxic and relatively nonirritant*

*CITRUS LIMON*

# Lemon

FAMILY: RUTACEAE

## Herbal/Folk Tradition

The juice and peel, high in vitamins A, B, and C, are widely used as a domestic seasoning. It was used for fever, such as malaria and typhoid, and employed for scurvy on English ships. The juice is invaluable for acidic disorders, rheumatism, and dysentery.

OUTER PEEL OF FRUIT

*A small evergreen tree up to 20ft (6m) high with serrated oval leaves, stiff thorns, and very fragrant flowers. The fruit turns from green to yellow on ripening.*

### DATAFILE

**AROMATHERAPY/ HOME USE**
See Lime, page 68.

**EXTRACTION**
Essential oil by cold expression from outer part of fresh peel.

**ACTIONS**
Anti-anemic, antimicrobial, antirheumatic, antisclerotic, antiscorbutic, antiseptic, antispasmodic, antitoxic, astringent, bactericidal, carminative, cicatrizant, depurative, diaphoretic, diuretic, febrifuge, hemostatic, hypotensive, insecticidal, rubefacient, stimulates white corpuscles, tonic, vermifuge.

**COMPATIBILITIES**
It blends well with citrus oils, lavender, orange blossom, ylang ylang, rose, sandalwood, olibanum, chamomile, benzoin, fennel, geranium, eyucalyputus, juniper, oakmoss, lavandin, elemi, labdanum.

### SAFETY DATA
*Nontoxic; may cause dermal irritation or sensitization reactions in some individuals – apply in moderation. Phototoxic – do not use on skin exposed to direct sunlight*

---

*CITRUS RETICULATA*

# Mandarin

FAMILY: RUTACEAE

## Herbal/Folk Tradition

In France it is regarded as a safe children's remedy for indigestion, hiccups, etc., and for the elderly since it helps strengthen the digestive function and liver.

OUTER PEEL OF FRUIT

YOUNG MANDARIN SHOOT

CUTTING WITH FLOWER BUDS

*A small evergreen tree up to 20ft (6m) high with glossy leaves, fragrant flowers, and bearing fleshy fruit. The tangerine is larger than the mandarin and rounder, with a yellower skin, more like the original Chinese type.*

### DATAFILE

**AROMATHERAPY/ HOME USE**
**Skin Care:** *Acne, blemishes, congested and oily skin, scars, stretch marks, toner.*
**Circulation, Muscles, and Joints:** *Fluid retention, obesity.*
**Digestive System:** *Digestive problems, dyspepsia, hiccoughs, intestinal problems.*
**Nervous System:** *Insomnia, nervous tension, restlessness. It is often used for children and pregnant women and is recommended in synergistic combinations with other citrus oils.*

**EXTRACTION**
Essential oil by cold expression from the outer peel. A mandarin petitgrain oil is produced in small quantities by steam distillation from the leaves and twigs.

**ACTIONS**
Antiseptic, antispasmodic, carminative, digestive, diuretic (mild), laxative (mild), sedative, stimulant (digestive and lymphatic), tonic.

**COMPATIBILITIES**
It blends well with citrus oils, especially orange blossom, and spice oils such as nutmeg.

### SAFETY DATA
*Nontoxic, nonirritant, nonsensitizing. Possibly phototoxic, although it has not been demonstrated decisively*

# Sweet orange

FAMILY: RUTACEAE

## Herbal/Folk Tradition

A very nutritious fruit, containing vitamins A, B, and C. In Chinese medicine the dried sweet

orange peel is used to treat coughs, colds, anorexia, and malignant breast sores. Li Shih-chên says: "The fruits of all the different species and varieties of citrus are considered by the Chinese to be cooling. The sweet varieties increase bronchial secretion and the sour promote expectoration. They all quench thirst, and are stomachic and carminative."[10]

*A yellowy-orange or dark orange mobile liquid with a sweet, fresh, fruity scent.*

*An evergreen tree, smaller than the bitter variety, less hardy with fewer or no spines. The fruit has a sweet pulp and nonbitter membranes.*

FRUIT PEEL

FRESH LEAVES

---

**DATAFILE**

### AROMATHERAPY/ HOME USE

**Skin Care:** *Oily skin, mouth ulcers.*
**Circulation, Muscles, and Joints:** *Obesity, palpitations, water retention.*
**Respiratory System:** *Bronchitis, chills.*
**Digestive System:** *Constipation, dyspepsia, spasm.*
**Immune System:** *Colds, flu.*
**Nervous System:** *Nervous tension and stress.*

### EXTRACTION

Essential oil by cold expression of the fresh ripe or almost ripe outer peel or by steam distillation of the fresh ripe or almost ripe outer peel. An inferior oil is also produced by distillation from the essences recovered as a by-product of orange juice manufacture.

### ACTIONS

Antidepressant, anti-inflammatory, antiseptic, bactericidal, carminative, choleretic, digestive, fungicidal, hypotensive, sedative , stimulant (digestive and lymphatic), stomachic, tonic.

### COMPATIBILITIES

Lavender, neroli, lemon, clary sage, myrrh, and spice oils, such as nutmeg and cinnamon.

*Citrus sinensis*

---

**SAFETY DATA**

*Generally nontoxic (although ingestion of large amounts of orange peel has been known to be fatal to children); distilled orange oil is phototoxic; its use on the skin should be avoided in direct sunlight. There is no evidence that expressed sweet orange oil is phototoxic, nonirritant and nonsensitizing (although limonene has caused dermatitis in a few individuals)*

*CITRUS X PARADISI*

# Grapefruit

FAMILY: RUTACEAE

### Herbal/Folk Tradition

It shares the nutritional qualities of other citrus species, being high in vitamin C and a valuable protection against infectious illness.

YOUNG FRUIT

FRUIT PEEL

*A cultivated tree, often over 33ft (10m) high with glossy leaves and large yellow fruits, believed to have derived from the shaddock (C. grandis).*

## DATAFILE

**AROMATHERAPY/ HOME USE**
**Skin Care:** *Acne, congested and oily skin, promotes hair growth, tones the skin and tissues.*
**Circulation, Muscles, and Joints:** *Cellulitis, exercise preparation, muscle fatigue, obesity, stiffness, water retention.*
**Immune System:** *Colds, flu.*
**Nervous System:** *Depression, headaches, nervous exhaustion, performance stress.*

**EXTRACTION**
Essential oil by cold expression from the fresh peel.

**ACTIONS**
Antiseptic, antitoxic, astringent, bactericidal, diuretic, depurative, stimulant (lymphatic, digestive), tonic.

**COMPATIBILITIES**
It blends well with lemon, palmarosa, bergamot, neroli, rosemary, cypress, lavender, geraniumn, cardomon, and other spice oils.

**SAFETY DATA**
Nontoxic, nonirritant, nonsensitizing, nonphototoxic.
It has a short shelf life – it oxidizes quickly

---

*COMMIPHORA ERYTHRAEA*

# Opopanax

FAMILY: BURSERACEAE

### Herbal/Folk Tradition

Opopanax, derived from *O. chironium,* has antispasmodic, expectorant, emmenagogue, and antiseptic properties, once used in asthma, hysteria, and visceral afflictions.

OPOPANAX GUM

*A tall tropical tree, similar to myrrh, which contains a natural oleogum resin in tubular vessels between the bark and wood of the trunk. The crude gum dries to form dark reddish-brown tear-shaped lumps.*

## DATAFILE

**AROMATHERAPY/ HOME USE**
Possibly similar uses to Myrrh, see page 74.

**EXTRACTION**
Essential oil by steam (or water) distillation from the crude oleogum resin. A resinoid by solvent extraction from the crude oleogum resin.

**ACTIONS**
Antiseptic, antispasmodic, balsamic, expectorant.

*Commiphora erythraea*

**COMPATIBILITIES**
It blends well with clary sage, cilantro, labdanum, bergamot, myrrh, frankincense, vetiver, sandalwood, patchouli, mimosa, fir needle, and neroli.

**SAFETY DATA**
Frequently adulterated – it is more expensive than the "hirabol myrrh".
The commercial resinoid is also usually mixed with a solvent such as myristate,
because it is otherwise unpourable at room temperatures

COMMIPHORA MYRRHA

# Myrrh

FAMILY: BURSERACEAE

CRUDE MYRRH

## Herbal/Folk Tradition

In China it is used for arthritis, menstrual problems, sores, and hemorrhoids. In the West it is considered to have an "opening, heating, drying nature" (Joseph Miller), good for asthma, coughs, common cold, catarrh, sore throat, weak gums and teeth, ulcers, and sores. It has also been used to treat leprosy. Current in the British Herbal Pharmacopoeia as a specific for mouth ulcers, gingivitis, and pharyngitis.

*The essential oil is a pale yellow to amber oily liquid with a warm, sweet-balsamic, slightly spicy medicinal odor.*

*The Commiphora species that yield myrrh are shrubs or small trees up to 33ft (10m) high, with knotted branches, trifolate aromatic leaves, and white flowers.*

---

**DATAFILE**

### AROMATHERAPY/ HOME USE

**Skin Care:** *Athlete's foot, chapped and cracked skin, eczema, mature complexions, ringworm, wounds, wrinkles.*

**Circulation, Muscles, and Joints:** *Arthritis.*

**Respiratory System:** *Asthma, bronchitis, catarrh, coughs, gum infections, gingivitis, mouth ulcers, sore throat, voice loss.*

**Digestive System:** *Diarrhea, dyspepsia, flatulence, hemorrhoids, loss of appetite.*

**Genitourinary System:** *Amenorrhea, leucorrhea, pruritis, thrush.*

**Immune System:** *Colds.*

### EXTRACTION

Resinoid (and resin absolute) by solvent extraction of the crude myrrh. Essential oil by steam distillation of the crude myrrh.

### ACTIONS

Anticatarrhal, anti-inflammatory, antimicrobial, antiphlogistic, antiseptic, astringent, balsamic, carminative, cicatrizant, emmenagogue, expectorant, fungicidal, revitalizing, sedative, stimulant (digestive, pulmonary), stomachic, tonic, uterine, vulnerary.

*Myrrh*

### COMPATIBILITIES

It blends well with frankincense, sandalwood, benzoin, oakmoss, cypress, juniper, mandarin, geranium, patchouli, thyme, mints, lavender, pine, and spices.

**SAFETY DATA**
*Nonirritant, nonsensitizing, possibly toxic in high concentration. Not to be used during pregnancy*

*COPAIFERA OFFICINALIS*

# Copaiba balsam

FAMILY: FABACEAE (LEGUMINOSAE)

### Herbal/Folk Tradition

Used for centuries in Europe in the treatment of chronic cystitis and bronchitis; also for treating piles, chronic diarrhea, and intestinal problems.

CRUDE COPAIBA BALSAM

*Wild-growing tropical tree up to 59ft (18m) high, with thick foliage and many branches. The natural oleoresin occurs as a physiological product from various Copaifera species. Not a "true" balsam.*

## DATAFILE

### AROMATHERAPY/ HOME USE

**Digestive System:** *Intestinal infections, piles.*
**Respiratory System:** *Bronchitis, chills, colds, coughs, etc.*
**Genitourinary System:** *Cystitis.*
**Nervous System:** *Stress-related conditions.*

### EXTRACTION

The crude balsam is collected by drilling holes into the tree trunks. An essential oil is obtained by dry distillation from the crude balsam.

### ACTIONS

Bactericidal, balsamic, disinfectant, diuretic, expectorant, stimulant.

### COMPATIBILITIES

The crude balsam blends well with styrax, amyris, lavandin, cedarwood, lavender, oakmoss, woods, and spices. The oil blends well with cananga, ylang ylang, vanilla, jasmine, violet, and other florals.

### SAFETY DATA
*Relatively nontoxic, nonirritant, possible sensitization. Large doses cause vomiting and diarrhea*

---

*CORIANDRUM SATIVUM*

# Cilantro

FAMILY: APIACEAE (UMBELLIFERAE)

### Herbal/Folk Tradition

The seeds and leaves are widely used as a garnish and domestic spice. It has also been used in the form of an infusion for children's diarrhea, digestive upsets, griping pains, anorexia, and flatulence.

CILANTRO SEEDS

*An aromatic annual herb about 3ft (1m) high with bright green delicate leaves, umbels of lacelike white flowers, followed by a mass of green (turning brown) round seeds.*

## DATAFILE

### AROMATHERAPY/ HOME USE

**Circulation, Muscles, and Joints:** *Accumulated fluids and toxins, arthritis, gout, muscular aches and pains, poor circulation, rheumatism, stiffness.*
**Digestive System:** *Anorexia, colic, diarrhea, dyspepsia, flatulence, nausea, piles, spasm.*
**Immune System:** *Colds, flu, infections (general), measles.*
**Nervous System:** *Debility, migraine, neuralgia, exhaustion.*

### EXTRACTION

Essential oil by steam distillation from the crushed ripe seeds.

### ACTIONS

Analgesic, aperitif, aphrodisiac, antioxidant, antirheumatic, antispasmodic, bactericidal, depurative, digestive, carminative, cytotoxic, fungicidal, larvicidal, lipolytic, revitalizing, stimulant (cardiac, circulatory, nervous system), stomachic.

### COMPATIBILITIES

It blends well with clary sage, bergamot, jasmine, olibanum, neroli, petitgrain, citronella, sandalwood, cypress, pine, ginger, cinnamon, and other spice oils.

### SAFETY DATA
*Generally nontoxic, nonirritant, nonsensitizing. Stupefying in large doses – use in moderation*

*CROTON ELEUTERIA*

# Cascarilla bark

FAMILY: EUPHORBIACEAE

### Herbal/Folk Tradition

The bark is used as an aromatic bitter and tonic for dyspepsia, diarrhea, dysentery, fever, debility, nausea, flatulence, vomiting, and chronic bronchitis. The leaves are used as a digestive tea and to flavor tobacco.

CASCARILLA BARK

*A large shrub or small tree up to 39ft (12m) high, with ovate silver-bronze leaves, pale yellowish-brown bark, and small white fragrant flowers. It bears fruits and flowers all year round.*

**AROMATHERAPY/ HOME USE**

**Respiratory System:** *Bronchitis, coughs.*

**Digestive System:** *Dyspepsia, flatulence, nausea.*

**Immune System:** *Flu.*

**EXTRACTION**

Essential oil by steam distillation from the dried bark (1.5–3 per cent yield).

**ACTIONS**

Astringent, antimicrobial, antiseptic, carminative, digestive, expectorant, stomachic, tonic.

**COMPATIBILITIES**

It blends well with nutmeg, pepper, pimento, sage, oakmoss, oriental and spicy bases.

**SAFETY DATA**
*Nonirritant, nonsensitizing, relatively nontoxic (possibly narcotic in large doses)*

---

*CUMINUM CYMINUM*

# Cumin

FAMILY: APIACEAE (UMBELLIFERAE)

### Herbal/Folk Tradition

A traditional Middle Eastern spice, and one of the main ingredients of curry. It is used in Ayurvedic medicine as a stimulant, especially for digestive problems such as colic, sluggish digestion, and dyspepsia.

CUMIN SEED

*A small, delicate, annual herb about 20in (50cm) high with a slender stem, dark green feathery leaves, and small pink or white flowers followed by small oblong seeds.*

**AROMATHERAPY/ HOME USE**

**Circulation, Muscles, and Joints:** *Accumulation of fluids or toxins, poor circulation.*

**Digestive System:** *Colic, dyspepsia, flatulence, indigestion, spasm.*

**Nervous System:** *Debility, headaches, migraine, nervous exhaustion.*

**EXTRACTION**

Essential oil by steam distillation from the ripe seeds.

**ACTIONS**

Antioxidant, antiseptic, antispasmodic, antitoxic, aphrodisiac, bactericidal, carminative, depurative, digestive, diuretic, emmenagogue, larvicidal, nervine, stimulant, tonic.

**COMPATIBILITIES**

It blends well with lavender, lavandin, rosemary, galbanum, rosewood, cardomon, and oriental-type fragrances.

**SAFETY DATA**
*Generally nontoxic, nonirritant, and nonsensitizing; however, the oil is phototoxic – do not expose treated skin to direct sunlight. Avoid during pregnancy*

*CUPRESSUS SEMPERVIRENS*

# Cypress
FAMILY: CUPRESSACEAE

## Herbal/Folk Tradition

Highly valued as a medicine and as an incense by ancient civilizations, it benefits the urinary system and is considered useful where there is excessive loss of fluid, such as heavy perspiration or menstrual loss and diarrhea.

FRESH CYPRESS

*A tall evergreen tree with slender branches and a statuesque conical shape. It bears small flowers and round, brownish-gray cones or nuts.*

### DATAFILE

**AROMATHERAPY/ HOME USE**

**Skin Care:** *Hemorrhoids, oily and overhydrated skin, excessive perspiration, insect repellent, pyorrhea (bleeding gums), varicose veins, wounds.*

**Circulation, Muscles, and Joints:** *Cellulitis, muscular cramp, edema, poor circulation, rheumatism.*

**Respiratory System:** *Asthma, bronchitis, coughing spasms.*

**Genitourinary System:** *Dysmenorrhea, menopausal problems, menorrhagia.*

**Nervous System:** *Nervous tension and stress.*

**EXTRACTION**
Essential oil by steam distillation from the needles, twigs, and, occasionally, cones.

**ACTIONS**
Antirheumatic, antiseptic, antispasmodic, astringent, deodorant, diuretic, hepatic, styptic, sudorific, tonic, vasoconstrictive.

**COMPATIBILITIES**
Cedarwood, pine, lavender, mandarin, clary sage, lemon, cardomon, juniper, Moroccan chamomile, orange ambrette seed, labdanum, benzoin, bergamot, and marjoram.

**SAFETY DATA**
*Nontoxic, nonirritant, and nonsensitizing*

---

*CURCUMA LONGA*

# Turmeric
FAMILY: ZINGIBERACEAE

## Herbal/Folk Tradition

A common spice, especially for curry powder. It is high in minerals and vitamins, especially vitamin C. It is widely used as a local home remedy. It was once used as a cure for jaundice.

TURMERIC ROOT

*A perennial tropical herb up to 3ft (1m) high, with a thick rhizome root, deep orange inside, lanceolate root leaves tapering at each end, and dull yellow flowers.*

### DATAFILE

**AROMATHERAPY/ HOME USE**

**Circulation, Muscles, and Joints:** *Arthritis, muscular aches and pains, rheumatism.*

**Digestive System:** *Anorexia, sluggish digestion, liver congestion.*

**EXTRACTION**
Essential oil by steam distillation from the "cured" rhizome. An oleoresin, absolute, and concrete are made by solvent extraction.

**ACTIONS**
Analgesic, antiarthritic, anti-inflammatory, antioxidant,

*Curcuma longa*

bactericidal, cholagogue, digestive, diuretic, hypotensive, insecticidal, laxative, rubefacient, stimulant.

**COMPATIBILITIES**
Cananga, labdanum, elecampane, ginger, orris, cassie, clary sage, and mimosa.

**SAFETY DATA**
*The ketone "tumerone" is moderately toxic and irritant in high concentration. Possible sensitization problems*

*CYMBOPOGON CITRATUS*

# Lemongrass

FAMILY: POACEAE (GRAMINEAE)

## Herbal/Folk Tradition

Employed in traditional Indian medicine for infectious illness and fever; modern research carried out in India shows that it also acts as a sedative on the central nervous system. It is also used as an insecticide and for food flavoring.

FRESH LEAVES

SLICED LEMONGRASS STEM

*A fast-growing, tall, aromatic perennial grass up to 5ft (1.5m) high, producing a network of roots and rootlets that rapidly exhaust the soil.*

### DATAFILE

**AROMATHERAPY/ HOME USE**

**Skin Care:** *Acne, athlete's foot, excessive perspiration, insect repellent (fleas, lice, ticks), open pores, pediculosis, scabies, tissue toner.*

**Circulation, Muscles, and Joints:** *Muscular pain, poor circulation and muscle tone, slack tissue.*

**Digestive System:** *Colitis, indigestion, gastroenteritis.*

**Immune System:** *Fevers, infectious disease.*

**Nervous System:** *Headaches, nervous exhaustion, and stress-related conditions.*

**EXTRACTION**

Essential oil by steam distillation from the fresh and partially dried leaves (grass), finely chopped.

**ACTIONS**

Analgesic, antidepressant, antimicrobial, antioxidant, antipyretic, antiseptic, astringent, bactericidal, carminative, deodorant, febrifuge, fungicidal, galactagogue, insecticidal, nervine, sedative (nervous), tonic.

**SAFETY DATA**

*Nontoxic, possible dermal irritation and/or sensitization in some individuals – use with care*

---

*CYMBOPOGON MARTINII VAR. MARTINII*

# Palmarosa

FAMILY: GRAMINACEAE

## Herbal/Folk Tradition

Formerly knwon as "Indian" or "Turkish" geranium oil, a term that dates back to the time when the oil was shipped from Bombay to the Red Sea and on to Constantinople and Bulgaria, where the oil was often used to adulterate rose oil.

DRIED PALMAROSA STEM

*A wild-growing herbaceous plant with long slender stems with terminal flowering tops and fragrant grassy leaves.*

### DATAFILE

**AROMATHERAPY/ HOME USE**

**Skin Care:** *Acne, dermatitis and minor skin infections, scars, sores, wrinkles; valuable for all types of treatment for the face, hands, feet, neck, and lips (moisturizes the skin, stimulates cellular regeneration, regulates sebum production).*

**Digestive System:** *Anorexia, digestive atonia, intestinal infections.*

**Nervous System:** *Nervous exhaustion, stress-related conditions.*

**EXTRACTION**

Essential oil by steam or water distillation of the fresh or dried grass.

**ACTIONS**

Antiseptic, bactericidal, cicatrizant, digestive, febrifuge, hydrating, stimulant (digestive, circulatory), tonic.

**COMPATIBILITIES**

It blends well with cananga, geranium, oakmoss, rosewood, amyris, sandalwood, guaiacwood, cedarwood, and floral oils.

**SAFETY DATA**

*Nontoxic, nonirritant, nonsensitizing*

*CYMBOPOGON NARDUS*

# Citronella

FAMILY: POACEAE (GRAMINEAE)

## Herbal/Folk Tradition

The leaves of citronella are used for their aromatic and medicinal value in many cultures, for fever, intestinal parasites, digestive and menstrual problems, as a stimulant, and an insect repellent. It is used in Chinese traditional medicine for rheumatic pain.

DRIED CITRONELLA

FRESH CITRONELLA GRASS

*A tall, aromatic, perennial grass, which has derived from the wild-growing "managrass" found in Sri Lanka.*

### DATAFILE

**AROMATHERAPY/
HOME USE**

**Skin Care:** *Excessive perspiration, oily skin, insect repellent. Mixed with cedarwood oil Virginia, it was a popular remedy against mosquito attacks before the advent of DDT and modern insecticides.*
**Immune System:** *Cold, flu, minor infections.*
**Nervous System:** *Fatigue, headaches, migraine, neuralgia.*

**EXTRACTION**
Essential oil by steam distillation of the fresh, part-dried, or dried grass.

**ACTIONS**
Antiseptic, antispasmodic, bactericidal, deodorant, diaphoretic, diuretic, emmenagogue, febrifuge, fungicidal, insecticide, stomachic, tonic, vermifuge.

**COMPATIBILITIES**
It blends well with geranium, lemon, bergamot, orange, cedarwood, and pine.

**SAFETY DATA**
*Nontoxic, nonirritant; may cause dermatitis in some individuals. Avoid during pregnancy*

---

*DAUCUS CAROTA*

# Carrot seed

FAMILY: APIACEAE (UMBELLIFERAE)

## Herbal/Folk Tradition

A highly nutritious plant, containing substantial amounts of vitamins A, C, B1, and B2. The seeds are used for treating the retention of urine, colic, kidney and digestive disorders, and to promote menstruation.

CARROT FRUIT (SEED)

*Annual or biennial herb with a 5-ft (1.5-m) high branched stem with hairy leaves and umbels of white lacy flowers.*

### DATAFILE

**AROMATHERAPY/
HOME USE**

**Skin Care:** *Dermatitis, eczema, psoriasis, rashes, revitalize, toning, mature complexions, wrinkles.*
**Circulation, Muscles, and Joints:** *Toxin accumulation, arthritis, gout, edema, rheumatism.*
**Digestive System:** *Anemia, anorexia, colic, indigestion, liver congestion.*
**Genitourinary and Endocrine Systems:** *Amenorrhea, dysmenorrhea, glandular problems, PMS.*

**EXTRACTION**
Essential oil by steam distillation from the dried fruit.

**ACTIONS**
Anthelmintic, antiseptic, carminative, depurative, diuretic, emmenagogue, hepatic, stimulant, tonic, vasodilatory, and smooth muscle relaxant.

**COMPATIBILITIES**
It blends well with costus, cassie, mimosa, cedarwood, geranium, citrus and spice oils.

**SAFETY DATA**
*Nontoxic, nonirritant, nonsensitizing*

*DIPTERYX ODORATA*

# Tonka

FAMILY: LEGUMINOSAE

## Herbal/Folk Tradition

In the Netherlands the fatty substance from the beans is sold as "taquin butter", which used to be used as an insecticide against moths in linen closets. The fluid extract has also been used in cases of whooping cough.

TONKA BEANS

*A very large tropical tree with big elliptical leaves and violet flowers, bearing fruit that contain a single black seed or "tonka bean," about the size of a lima bean. The beans are collected and dried and soaked in alcohol or rum to make them swell.*

### DATAFILE

**AROMATHERAPY/ HOME USE**
None.

**EXTRACTION**
A concrete and absolute by solvent extraction from the "cured" beans.

**ACTIONS**
Insecticidal, narcotic, tonic (cardiac).

**COMPATIBILITIES**
It blends well with lavender, lavandin, clary sage, styrax, bergamot, oakmoss, helichrysum, and citronella.

#### SAFETY DATA
*Oral and dermal toxin, due to high coumarin content*

---

*ELETTARIA CARDAMOMUM*

# Cardomon

FAMILY: ZINGIBERACEAE

## Herbal/Folk Tradition

Used extensively as a domestic spice. It has been used in traditional Chinese and Indian medicine for over 3,000 years, especially for pulmonary disease, fever, digestive and urinary complaints.

CARDOMON SEEDS

*A perennial, reedlike herb up to 13ft (4m) high, with long, silk blade-shaped leaves. Its long sheathing stems bear small yellowish flowers with purple tips, followed by oblong red-brown seeds.*

### DATAFILE

**AROMATHERAPY/ HOME USE**
**Digestive System:** *Anorexia, colic, cramp, dyspepsia, flatulence, griping pains, halitosis, heartburn, indigestion, vomiting.*
**Nervous System:** *Mental fatigue, nervous strain.*

**EXTRACTION**
Essential oil by steam distillation from the dried ripe fruit (seeds). An oleoresin is also produced in small quantities.

**ACTIONS**
Antiseptic, antispasmodic, aphrodisiac, carminative, cephalic, digestive, diuretic, sialagogue, stimulant, stomachic, tonic (nerve).

**COMPATIBILITIES**
It blends well with rose, olibanum, orange, bergamot, cinnamon, cloves, caraway, ylang ylang, labdanum, cedarwood, orange blossom, and oriental bases in general.

#### SAFETY DATA
*Nontoxic, nonirritant, nonsensitizing*

# Borneol

FAMILY: DIPTEROCARPACEAE

CRYSTALLIZED BORNEOL

### Herbal/Folk Tradition

Borneol has long been regarded as a panacea by many Eastern civilizations, especially in ancient Persia, India, and China. It was used as a powerful remedy against plague and other infectious diseases, stomach and bowel complaints. In China it was also used for embalming purposes. "It is mentioned by Marco Polo in the thirteenth century and Camoens in 1571 who called it the 'balsam of disease.'"[11] It is valued for ceremonial purposes in the East generally, and in China particularly for funeral rites. Its odor repels insects and ants, and it is therefore highly regarded as lumber for the construction of buildings.

*The camphora tree grows to a great height, a majestic tree often over 82ft (25m) high, with a thick trunk up to 6ft (2m) in diameter. Borneol is a natural exudation found beneath the bark in crevices and fissures of some mature trees (about 1 per cent); young trees produce only a clear yellow liquid known as "liquid camphor".*

## DATAFILE

### AROMATHERAPY HOME USE

**Skin Care:** *Cuts, bruises, insect repellent.*

**Circulation, Muscles, and Joints:** *Debility, poor circulation, rheumatism, sprains.*

**Respiratory System:** *Bronchitis, coughs.*

**Immune System:** *Colds, fever, flu, and other infectious diseases.*

**Nervous System:** *Nervous exhaustion, stress-related conditions, neuralgia.*

### EXTRACTION

The borneol is collected from the tree trunk in its crude crystalline form (the locals test each tree first by making incisions in the trunk to detect its presence). The so-called oil of borneol is extracted by steam distillation of the wood.

### ACTIONS

Mildly analgesic, antidepressant, antiseptic, antispasmodic, antiviral, carminative, rubefacient, stimulant of the adrenal cortex, tonic (cardiac and general).

*Dryobalanops aromatica*

### SAFETY DATA

*Nontoxic, nonsensitizing, dermal irritant in concentration*

# Lemon-scented eucalyptus

FAMILY: MYRTACEAE

## Herbal/Folk Tradition

Used traditionally for perfuming the linen closet by enclosing the dried leaves in a small sachet. During the last century it was seen as a good insect repellent, especially for cockroaches and silverfish.

SEEDS

DRIED LEAVES

*A tall evergreen tree with a smooth dimpled bark, blotched in gray, cream, and pink. The young leaves are oval, the mature leaves narrow and tapering.*

### DATAFILE

**AROMATHERAPY/HOME USE**

Not compatible with homeopathic treatment.

**Skin Care:** *Athlete's foot and other fungal infections (e.g. candida), cuts, dandruff, herpes, insect repellent, scabs, sores, wounds.*

**Respiratory System:** *Asthma, laryngitis, sore throat.*

**Immune System:** *Colds, fevers, infectious skin conditions such as chickenpox, infectious disease.*

**EXTRACTION**

Essential oil by steam distillation from the leaves and twigs.

**ACTIONS**

Antiseptic, antiviral, bactericidal, deodorant, expectorant, fungicidal, insecticide.

**SAFETY DATA**

Nontoxic, nonirritant, possible sensitization in some individuals. Eucalyptus oil is toxic when taken internally – see blue gum eucalyptus.

---

# Broad-leaved peppermint eucalyptus

FAMILY: MYRTACEAE

## Herbal/Folk Tradition

The Aborigines used the burning leaves in the form of a fumigation for the relief of fever: "heat went out of sick man and into fire."

SEEDS

DRIED LEAVES

*A robust, medium-size eucalyptus tree, with a short trunk, spreading branches and fibrous gray bark. The young leaves are blue and heart-shaped, the mature leaves are very aromatic, thick, and tapering at both ends.*

### DATAFILE

**AROMATHERAPY/HOME USE**

Not compatible with homeopathic treatment.

**Skin Care:** *Cuts, sores, ulcers, etc.*

**Circulation, Muscles, and Joints:** *Arthritis, muscular aches and pains, rheumatism, sports injuries, sprains,*

**Respiratory System:** *Asthma, bronchitis, catarrh, coughs, throat and mouth infection.*

**Immune System:** *Colds, fevers, flu, infectious illnesses, e.g. measles.*

**Nervous System:** *Headaches, nervous exhaustion, neuralgia, sciatica.*

**EXTRACTION**

Essential oil by steam distillation from the leaves and twigs.

**ACTIONS**

Analgesic, antineuralgic, antirheumatic, antiseptic, antispasmodic, antiviral, balsamic, cicatrizant, decongestant, deodorant, depurative, diuretic, expectorant, febrifuge, hypoglycemic, parasiticide, prophylactic, rubefacient, stimulant, vermifuge, vulnerary.

**SAFETY DATA**

Nontoxic, nonirritant (in dilution), nonsensitizing. Eucalyptus oil is toxic if taken internally, see blue gum eucalyptus page 83

*EUCALYPTUS GLOBULUS VAR. GLOBULUS*

# Blue gum eucalyptus

FAMILY: MYRTACEAE *LAVANDULA ANGUSTIFOLIA*

## Herbal/Folk Tradition

A traditional household remedy in Australia, the leaves and oil are used especially for respiratory ailments such as bronchitis and croup, and the dried leaves are smoked like tobacco for asthma. It is also used for feverish conditions (malaria, typhoid, cholera, etc.) and skin problems such as burns, ulcers, and wounds. Aqueous extracts are used for aching joints, bacterial dysentery, ringworms, tuberculosis, etc. and employed for similar reasons in Western and Eastern medicine. The wood is also used for lumber production in Spain.

FRESH LEAVES

*A beautiful, tall, evergreen tree, up to 295ft (90m) high. The young trees have bluish-green oval leaves while the mature trees develop long, narrow, yellowish leaves, creamy-white flowers, and a smooth, pale gray bark often covered with a white powder.*

**DATAFILE**

### AROMATHERAPY/ HOME USE

Not compatible with homeopathic treatment.

**Skin Care:** *Burns, blisters, cuts, herpes, insect bites, insect repellent, lice, skin infections, wounds.*

**Circulation, Muscles, and Joints:** *Muscular aches and pains, poor circulation, rheumatoid arthritis, sprains, etc.*

**Respiratory System:** *Asthma, bronchitis, catarrh, coughs, sinusitis, throat infections.*

**Genitourinary System:** *Cystitis, leucorrhea.*

**Immune System:** *Chickenpox, colds, epidemics, flu, measles.*

**Nervous System:** *Debility, headaches, neuralgia.*

### EXTRACTION

Essential oil by steam distillation from the fresh or partially dried leaves and young twigs.

### ACTIONS

See Broad-leaved peppermint eucalyptus, page 82.

### COMPATIBILITIES

It blends well with thyme, rosemary, lavender, marjoram, pine, cedarwood, and lemon.

*Eucalyptus globulus var. globulus*

**SAFETY DATA**

*Externally nontoxic, nonirritant (in dilution), nonsensitizing. "When taken internally eucalyptus oil is toxic and as little as 3.5ml has been reported as fatal."[2]*

# Oakmoss

FAMILY: USNEACEAE

### Herbal/Folk Tradition

*Sticta pulmonaceae*, a greeny-brown lichen frequently harvested along with *E. prunastri*, is also called oak lungs, lung moss, lungwort, or "lungs of oak" by the Native Americans who use it for respiratory complaints and for treating wounds.

OAK BARK

OAKMOSS LICHEN

*A light green lichen found growing primarily on oak trees, sometimes on other species.*

DATAFILE

**AROMATHERAPY/ HOME USE**
As a fixative.

**EXTRACTION**
A range of products is produced: a concrete and an absolute by solvent extraction from the lichen that has often been soaked in lukewarm water prior to extraction; an absolute oil by vacuum distillation of the concrete; resins and resinoids by alcohol extraction of the raw material. Most important of these products is the absolute.

**ACTIONS**
Antiseptic, demulcent, expectorant, fixative.

**COMPATIBILITIES**
The concrete, resin, and resinoids have a high fixative value and blend with virtually all other oils: they are extensively used in perfumery to lend body and rich natural undertones to all perfume types.

**SAFETY DATA**
*Extensively compounded or bouqueted by cutting or adulteration with other lichen or synthetic perfume materials*

# Asafetida

FAMILY: APIACEAE (UMBELLIFERAE)

### Herbal/Folk Tradition

Reputed to treat various ailments including asthma, bronchitis, coughs, convulsions, constipation, flatulence, and hysteria. In Chinese medicine it is used to treat neurasthenia.

FRESH ASAFETIDA

*A large branching perennial herb up to 10ft (3m) high, with a thick fleshy root system and pale yellow-green flowers.*

DATAFILE

**AROMATHERAPY/ HOME USE**
Respiratory System:
*"There is evidence that the volatile oil is expelled through the lungs, therefore it is excellent for asthma, bronchitis, whooping cough, etc."[13]*
Nervous System:
*Fatigue, nervous exhaustion, and stress-related conditions.*

**EXTRACTION**
The oleoresin is obtained by making incisions into the root and plant. The juice leaks and harden into dark reddish lumps, before being collected. The essential oil is obtained from the resin by steam distillation.

**ACTIONS**
Antispasmodic, carminative, expectorant, hypotensive, stimulant.

**SAFETY DATA**
*Available information indicates the oil to be relatively nontoxic and nonirritant. However, it has the reputation for being the most adulterated "drug" on the market. Before being sold, the oleoresin is often mixed with red clay or similar substitutes*

*FERULA GALBANIFLUA*

# Galbanum

FAMILY: APIACEAE (UMBELLIFERAE)

## Herbal/Folk Tradition

It was used by the ancient civilizations as an incense, and in Egypt for cosmetics and in the embalming process. It is generally used in the East in a similar way to asafetida: for treating wounds, inflammations, and skin disorders and also for respiratory, digestive, and nervous complaints. Zalou root (*F. hermonic*) is used in Beirut as an aphrodisiac.

GALBANUM FLOWERS

FRESH LEAVES

*A colorless, or pale yellow or olive liquid with a fresh green top note and woody-dry balsamic undertone.*

*A large perennial herb with a smooth stem, shiny leaflets, and small flowers. It contains resin ducts that exude a milky juice, a natural oleoresin. The dried resinous exudation is collected by making incisions at the base of the stem.*

---

**DATAFILE**

### AROMATHERAPY/ HOME USE

**Skin Care:** *Abscesses, acne, boils, cuts, heals scar tissue, inflammations, tones the skin, mature skin, wrinkles, wounds – "signifies drying and preservation."*[14]

**Circulation, Muscles, and Joints:** *Poor circulation, muscular aches and pains, rheumatism.*

**Respiratory System:** *Asthma, bronchitis, catarrh, chronic coughs.*

**Digestive System:** *Cramp, flatulence, indigestion.*

**Nervous System:** *Nervous tension and stress-related complaints.*

### EXTRACTION

Essential oil by water or steam distillation from the oleoresin or gum – only the Levant or soft type is used for oil production. A partially deterpenized oil is produced, known as "galbanol".

### ACTIONS

Analgesic, anti-inflammatory, antimicrobial, antiseptic, antispasmodic, aphrodisiac, balsamic, carminative, cicatrizant, digestive, diuretic, emmenagogue, expectorant, hypotensive, restorative, tonic.

*Ferula galbaniflua*

### COMPATIBILITIES

Hyacinth, violet, narcissus, lavender, geranium, oakmoss, opopanax, pine, fir, styrax, and oriental bases.

---

**SAFETY DATA**

*Nontoxic, nonirritant, nonsensitizing*

*FOENICULUM VULGARE*

# Fennel

FAMILY: APIACEAE (UMBELLIFERAE)

FENNEL SEEDS

## Herbal/Folk Tradition

A herb of ancient medical repute, believed to convey longevity, courage, and strength. It was also used to

ward off evil spirits, strengthen the eyesight, and neutralize poisons. It is considered good for obstructions of the liver, spleen, and gall bladder and for digestive complaints. It has traditionally been used for obesity, which may be due to a type of estrogenic action, which also increases the milk of nursing mothers. Still current in the British Herbal Pharmacopoeia, used locally for conjunctivitis, blepharitis, and pharyngitis.

*Biennial or perennial herb up to 6ft (2m) high, with feathery leaves and golden yellow flowers. There are two main varieties of fennel: bitter or common fennel, slightly taller with less divided leaves occurring in a cultivated or wild form; and sweet fennel (also known as Roman, garden, or French fennel), which is always cultivated.*

FRESH FENNEL LEAVES

### DATAFILE

#### AROMATHERAPY/HOME USE
Bitter fennel: *none.*
Sweet fennel:
Skin Care: *Bruises, dull, oily, mature complexions, pyorrhea.*
Circulation, Muscles, and Joints: *Cellulitis, obesity, edema, rheumatism.*
Respiratory System: *Asthma, bronchitis.*
Digestive System: *Anorexia, colic, constipation, dyspepsia, flatulence, hiccough, nausea.*
Genitourinary System: *Amenorrhea, insufficient milk (in nursing mothers), menopausal problems.*

#### EXTRACTION
Essential oil by steam distillation. Sweet fennel oil is made from crushed seeds, and bitter fennel oil from crushed seeds or the whole herb (the wild "weed").

#### ACTIONS
Aperitif, anti-inflammatory, antimicrobial, antiseptic, antispasmodic, carminative, depurative, diuretic, emmenagogue, expectorant, galactagogue, laxative, orexigenic, stimulant (circulatory), splenic, stomachic, tonic, vermifuge.

*Foeniculum vulgare*

#### COMPATIBILITIES
Sweet fennel oil blends well with geranium, lavender, rose, and sandalwood.

#### SAFETY DATA
*Nonirritant, relatively nontoxic, narcotic in large doses; bitter fennel may cause sensitization. Bitter fennel oil should not be used on the skin at all, although it is considered superior medicinally. Neither oil should be used by epileptics or during pregnancy. Use in moderation*

*GARDENIA JASMINOIDES*

# Gardenia

FAMILY: RUBIACEAE

## Herbal/Folk Tradition

The flowers are used locally to flavor tea, much like jasmine.

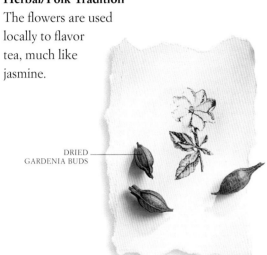

DRIED GARDENIA BUDS

*A decorative bush, often grown for ornamental purposes, bearing fragrant white flowers.*

DATAFILE

**AROMATHERAPY/ HOME USE**
Perfume.

**EXTRACTION**
An absolute (and concrete) by solvent extraction from the fresh flowers.

**ACTIONS**
Antiseptic, aphrodisiac.

**COMPATIBILITIES**
It blends well with ylang ylang, jasmine, tuberose, orange blossom, rose, spice and citrus oils

*Gardenia jasminoides* Native to the Far East, India, and China. Efforts to produce the oil commercially have been largely unsuccessful.

**SAFETY DATA**
*Safety data unavailable at present. Almost all gardenia oil is now synthetically produced*

---

*GAULTHERIA PROCUMBENS*

# Wintergreen

FAMILY: ERICACEAE

## Herbal/Folk Tradition

The plant has been used for respiratory conditions such as chronic mucus discharge, but is employed mainly for joint and muscular problems such as lumbago, sciatica, neuralgia.

FRESH WINTERGREEN

*A small evergreen herb up to 6in (15cm) high with slender creeping stems shooting forth erect twigs with leathery serrated leaves and drooping white flowers, which are followed by fleshy scarlet berries.*

**DATAFILE**

**AROMATHERAPY/ HOME USE**
None. Avoid use, both internally and externally.

**EXTRACTION**
Essential oil by steam (or water) distillation from the leaf, previously macerated in warm water.

**ACTIONS**
Analgestic (mild), anti-inflammatory, antirheumatic, antitussive, astringent, carminative, diuretic, emmenagogue, galactagogue, stimulant.

**COMPATIBILITIES**
It blends well with oregano, mints, thyme, ylang ylang, narcissus, and vanilla.

**SAFETY DATA**
*Toxic, irritant, and sensitizing – an environmental hazard or marine pollutant. The true oil is almost obsolete, having been replaced by synthetic methyl salicylate. See also Sweet birch oil, page 55*

*HUMULUS LUPULUS*

# Hops

FAMILY: MORACEAE

## Herbal/Folk Tradition

Best known as a nerve remedy, for insomnia, nervous tension, neuralgia, and also for sexual neurosis in both sexes. It supports the female estrogens and is useful for amenorrhea (absence of periods). It also acts as a mild sedative, commonly used in the form of the hop pillow where the heavy aromatic odor has been shown to relax by direct action at the olfactory centers. It has also been used for heart disease, and stomach and liver complaints, including bacterial dysentery.

In China it is used for pulmonary tuberculosis and cystitis. It is used to make beer. Current in the British Herbal Pharmacopoeia as a specific for restlessness with nervous headaches and/or indigestion.

DRIED HOPS

*Perennial creeping, twining herb up to 26ft (8m) high, which bears male and female flowers on separate plants. It has dark green, heart-shaped leaves and greeny-yellow flowers. A volatile oil, called lupulin, is formed in the glandular hairs of the cones or "strobiles".*

## DATAFILE

### AROMATHERAPY/HOME USE

**Skin Care:** *Dermatitis, rashes, rough skin, ulcers.*
**Respiratory System:** *Asthma, spasmodic cough.*
**Digestive System:** *Indigestion, nervous dyspepsia.*
**Genitourinary and Endocrine Systems:** *Amenorrhea, menstrual cramp, supports female estrogens, promotes feminine characteristics, reduces sexual overactivity.*
**Nervous System:** *Headaches, insomnia, nervous tension, neuralgia, stress-related conditions.*

### EXTRACTION

Essential oil by steam distillation from the dried cones or catkins, known as "strobiles". (An absolute is also produced by solvent extraction for perfumery use.)

### ACTIONS

Anodyne, an aphrodisiac, antimicrobial, antiseptic, antispasmodic, astringent, bactericidal, carminative, diuretic, emollient, estrogenic properties, hypnotic, nervine, sedative, soporific.

*Humulus lupulus*

### COMPATIBILITIES

It blends well with pine, hyacinth, nutmeg, copaiba, balsam, citrus, and spice oils.

### SAFETY DATA

*Generally nontoxic (narcotic in excessive amounts) and nonirritant; may cause sensitization in some individuals. Should be avoided by those suffering from depression*

# Helichrysum

FAMILY: ASTERACEAE (COMPOSITAE)

### Herbal/Folk Tradition

In Europe it is used for respiratory ailments such as asthma, whooping cough, and chronic bronchitis; also for headaches, migraine, liver ailments, and skin complaints including allergies and psoriasis.

FRESH LEAVES

*An aromatic herb, up to 24in (60cm) high with a branched stem and woody base. The brightly colored, daisylike flowers become dry as the plant matures, yet retain their color.*

## DATAFILE

**AROMATHERAPY/ HOME USE**

**Skin Care:** *Abscess, acne, allergic conditions, blemishes, boils, burns, cuts, dermatitis, eczema, inflammation, wounds.*

**Circulation, Muscles, and Joints:** *Muscular aches and pains, sprains, strains, rheumatism.*

**Respiratory System:** *Asthma, bronchitis, chronic coughs.*

**Digestive System:** *Liver congestion, spleen congestion.*

**Immune System:** *Bacterial infections, colds, flu, fever.*

**Nervous System:** *Depression, debility, lethargy, neuralgia.*

**EXTRACTION**

Essential oil by steam distillation from fresh flowers, absolute by solvent extraction.

**ACTIONS**

Antiallergenic, anti-inflammatory, antimicrobial, antitussive, antiseptic, astringent, cholagogue, cicatrizant, diuretic, hepatic, expectorant, fungicidal, nervine.

**COMPATIBILITIES**

Citrus oils, chamomile, clove, boronia, labdanum, lavender, mimosa, oakmoss, geranium, clary sage, rose, Peru balsam.

**SAFETY DATA**
*Nontoxic, nonirritant, nonsensitizing*

---

# Hyacinth

FAMILY: LILIACEAE

### Herbal/Folk Tradition

The wild bulbs are poisonous; however, the white juice used to be employed as a substitute for starch or glue. The dried and powdered roots, are balsamic, and believed to have some styptic properties.

SLICED HYACINTH BULB

*A much-loved cultivated plant with fragrant, bell-shaped flowers of many colors, bright lance-shaped leaves, and a round bulb.*

## DATAFILE

**AROMATHERAPY/ HOME USE**

**Nervous System:**
*The Greeks described the fragrance of hyacinth as being refreshing and invigorating to a tired mind. It may also be used for stress-related conditions, in self-hypnosis techniques, and in the development of the creative right-hand side of the brain.*

**EXTRACTION**

Concrete and absolute by solvent extraction from the flowers. (An essential oil is also obtained by steam distillation from the absolute.)

**ACTIONS**

Antiseptic, balsamic, hypnotic, sedative, styptic.

**COMPATIBILITIES**

It blends well with narcissus, violet, ylang ylang, styrax, galbanum, jasmine, neroli, and with oriental-type bases.

**SAFETY DATA**
*No safety data available at present. Most commercial hyacinth is nowadays adulterated or synthetic*

*HYSSOPUS OFFICINALIS*

# Hyssop

FAMILY: LAMIACEAE (LABIATAE)

## Herbal/Folk Tradition

*H. officinalis* has an ancient medical reputation and was used for purifying sacred places and employed as a strewing herb.

It is used mainly for respiratory and digestive complaints, and externally for rheumatism, bruises, sores, earache, and toothache.

FRESH HYSSOP

*An attractive perennial, almost evergreen subshrub up to 24in (60cm) high with a woody stem, small, lance-shaped leaves, and purplish-blue flowers.*

### DATAFILE

**AROMATHERAPY/ HOME USE**

**Skin Care:** *Bruises, cuts, dermatitis, eczema, inflammation, wounds.*

**Circulation, Muscles, and Joints:** *Low or high blood pressure, rheumatism.*

**Respiratory System:** *Asthma, bronchitis, catarrh, cough, sore throat, tonsillitis.*

**Digestive System:** *Colic, indigestion.*

**Genitourinary System:** *Amenorrhea, leucorrhea.*

**Immune System:** *Colds, flu.*

**Nervous System:** *Anxiety, fatigue.*

**EXTRACTION**

Essential oil by steam distillation from leaves and flowering tops.

**ACTIONS**

Astringent, antiseptic, antispasmodic, antiviral, bactericidal, carminative, cephalic, cicatrizant, digestive, diuretic, emmenagogue, expectorant, febrifuge, hypertensive, nervine, sedative, sudorific, tonic (heart), vermifuge, vulnerary.

**COMPATIBILITIES**

Bay leaf, citrus, clary sage, geranium, myrtle, and rosemary.

### SAFETY DATA

*Nonirritant, nonsensitizing; the oil is moderately toxic due to the pinocamphone content. To be used only in moderation and avoided in pregnancy and by epileptics. Contraindicated in cases of high blood pressure*

---

*ILLICIUM VERUM*

# Star anise

FAMILY: ILLICIACEAE

## Herbal/Folk Tradition

Used in Chinese medicine for over 1,300 years for its stimulating effect on the digestive system and for respiratory disorders such as bronchitis and dry coughs.

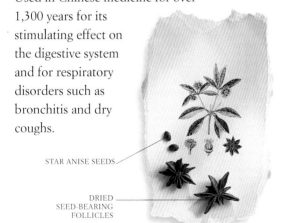

STAR ANISE SEEDS

DRIED SEED-BEARING FOLLICLES

*Evergreen tree up to 39ft (12m) high with a tall, slender white trunk. It bears fruit that consist of five to thirteen seed-bearing follicles attached to a central axis in the shape of a star.*

### DATAFILE

**AROMATHERAPY/ HOME USE**

**Circulation, Muscles, and Joints:** *Muscular aches and pains, rheumatism.*

**Respiratory System:** *Bronchitis, coughs.*

**Digestive System:** *Colic, cramp, flatulence, indigestion.*

**Immune System:** *Colds.*

**EXTRACTION**

Essential oil by steam distillation from the fruits, fresh or partially dried. An oil is also produced from leaves in small quantities.

**ACTIONS**

Antiseptic, carminative, expectorant, insect repellent, stimulant.

**COMPATIBILITIES**

It blends well with rose, lavender, orange, pine, and other spice oils, and has excellent masking properties.

### SAFETY DATA

*Despite the anethole content, it does not appear to be a dermal irritant, unlike aniseed. In large doses it is narcotic and slows down the circulation; it can lead to cerebral disorders. Use in moderation only. Avoid during pregnancy*

*INULA HELENIUM*

# Elecampane

FAMILY: ASTERACEAE (COMPOSITAE)

## Herbal/Folk Tradition

An herb that used to be candied and sold as a sweetmeat. It is used for respiratory conditions such as bronchitis, asthma, and whooping cough, disorders of the digestion, intestines, and gall bladder

FRESH
ELECAMPANE

*A perennial herb up to 5ft (1.5m) high, with a stout stem covered with soft hairs. It has oval pointed leaves with a velvety underside, yellow flowers, and fleshy rhizome roots.*

### DATAFILE

**AROMATHERAPY/
HOME USE**
None. NB: Elecampane is a rich source of inulin. Sweet inulin oil is said to have sedative, anti-inflammatory, hyperthermic, cardioregulative, diuretic, and depurative actions. When it is used as an inhalation or by aerosol treatment this variety of Inula avoids the sensitization problems of elecampane, .

**EXTRACTION**
Essential oil by steam distillation from dried roots and rhizomes.

**ACTIONS**
Alterative, anthelmintic, anti-inflammatory, antiseptic, antispasmodic, antitussive, astringent, bactericidal, diaphoretic, diuretic, expectorant, fungicidal, hyperglycemic, hypotensive, stomachic, tonic.

**COMPATIBILITIES**
It blends well with cananga, cinnamon, labdanum, lavender, mimosa, frankincense, orris, tuberose, volet, cedarwood, patchouli, sandalwood, cypress, bergamot, and oriental fragrances.

### SAFETY DATA
*Nontoxic, nonirritant, a severe dermal sensitizer. In clinical tests it caused "extremely severe allergic reactions" in 23 out of 25 volunteers; therefore, it is recommended that the oil "should not be used on the skin at all"[15]*

---

*IRIS PALLIDA*

# Orris

FAMILY: IRIDACEAE

## Herbal/Folk Tradition

In ancient Greece and Rome orris root was used extensively in perfumery, and its medicinal qualities were held in high esteem. It was once used for upper respiratory tract catarrh, coughs, and for diarrhea in infants.

ORRIS ROOT

*A decorative perennial plant up to 5ft (1.5m) high, with sword-shaped leaves, a creeping fleshy rootstock, and delicate, scented, pale blue flowers.*

### DATAFILE

**AROMATHERAPY/
HOME USE**
None. However, the powdered orris, which is a common article, may be used as a dry shampoo, a body powder, a fixative for pot-pourris, and to scent linen.

**EXTRACTION**
A concrete is produced by steam distillation from the rhizomes that have been peeled, washed, dried, and pulverized. Rhizomes must be stored for at least three years otherwise they have virtually no scent. An absolute is produced by alkali washing in ethyl ether solution to remove the myristic acid from the concrete oil. A resin or resinoid is produced by alcohol extraction from the peeled rhizomes.

**ACTIONS**
Dried root – antidiarrheal, demulcent, expectorant. Fresh root – diuretic, cathartic, emetic.

**COMPATIBILITIES**
It blends well with cedarwood, sandalwood, vetiver, cypress, mimosa, labdanum, bergamot, clary sage, rose, violet and other florals.

### SAFETY DATA
*The fresh root causes nausea and vomiting in large doses. The oil and absolute are much adulterated or synthetic – "true" orris absolute is three times the price of jasmine*

*JASMINUM OFFICINALE*

# Jasmine

FAMILY: OLEACEAE

FRESH JASMINE

## Herbal/Folk Tradition

In China the flowers of *J. officinale var. grandiflorum* are used to treat hepatitis, liver cirrhosis, and dysentery; the flowers of *J. sambac* are used for conjunctivitis, dysentery, skin ulcers, and tumors. The root is used to treat headaches, insomnia, pain due to dislocated joints and rheumatism.

In the West, the common jasmine was said in Culpeper's *Complete Herbal* to "warm the womb … and facilitate the birth; it is useful for cough, difficulty of breathing, etc. It disperses crude humours, and is good for cold and catarrhous constitutions, but not for the hot."[16] It was also used for hard, contracted limbs and problems with the nervous and reproductive systems.

*An evergreen shrub or vine up to 33ft (10m) high with delicate, bright green leaves and star-shaped very fragrant white flowers.*

---

### DATAFILE

**AROMATHERAPY/ HOME USE**

**Skin Care:** *Dry, greasy, irritated, sensitive skin.*

**Circulation, Muscles, and Joints:** *Muscular spasm, sprains.*

**Respiratory System:** *Catarrh, coughs, hoarseness, laryngitis.*

**Genitourinary System:** *Dysmenorrhea, frigidity, labor pains, uterine disorders.*

**Nervous System:** *Depression, nervous exhaustion and stress-related conditions. "It … produces a feeling of optimism, confidence and euphoria. It is most useful in cases where there is apathy, indifference, or listlessness."[17]*

**EXTRACTION**

A concrete is produced by solvent extraction; the absolute is obtained from the concrete by separation with alcohol. An essential oil is produced by steam distillation of the absolute.

**ACTIONS**

Analgesic (mild), antidepressant, anti-inflammatory, antiseptic, antispasmodic, aphrodisiac, carminative, cicatrizant, expectorant, galactagogue, parturient, sedative, tonic (uterine).

*Jasminum officinale*

**COMPATIBILITIES**

It blends well with rose, sandalwood, clary sage, and all the citrus oils. It has the ability to round off any rough notes and blend with virtually everything.

---

### SAFETY DATA

*Nontoxic, nonirritant, generally nonsensitizing (an allergic reaction has been known to occur in some individuals)*

*JUNIPERUS ASHEI*

# Texas cedarwood

FAMILY: CUPRESSACEAE

## Herbal/Folk Tradition

In New Mexico the Native Americans use cedarwood oil for skin rashes. It is also used for arthritis and rheumatism.

TEXAS CEDARWOOD CHIPPINGS

*A small, alpine evergreen tree up to 23ft (7m) high with stiff green needles and an irregular-shaped trunk and branches, which tend to be crooked or twisted. The wood also tends to crack easily, so it is not used for lumber.*

### DATAFILE

**AROMATHERAPY/ HOME USE**

**Skin Care:** *Acne, dandruff, eczema, greasy hair, insect repellent, oily skin, psoriasis.*

**Circulation, Muscles, and Joints:** *Arthritis, rheumatism.*

**Respiratory System:** *Bronchitis, catarrh, congestion, coughs, sinusitis.*

**Genitourinary System:** *Cystitis, leucorrhea.*

**Nervous System:** *Nervous tension and stress-related disorders.*

**EXTRACTION**

Essential oil by steam distillation from the heartwood and wood shavings, etc.

**ACTIONS**

Antiseptic, antispasmodic, astringent, diuretic, expectorant, sedative (nervous), stimulant (circulatory).

**COMPATIBILITIES**

Rectified oil blends well with patchouli, spruce, vetiver, pine, and leather-type scents.

**SAFETY DATA**

*Externally the oil is relatively nontoxic; it can cause acute local irritation and possible sensitization in some. Use in dilution only with care, in moderation. Avoid during pregnancy. Generally safer to use Atlas cedarwood*

---

*JUNIPERUS COMMUNIS*

# Juniper

FAMILY: CUPRESSACEAE

## Herbal/Folk Tradition

Used medicinally for urinary infections, for respiratory problems, as well as gastrointestinal infections and worms. It helps expel the buildup of uric acid in the joints and is employed in gout, rheumatism, and arthritis.

FLOWERS

BARK AND NEEDLES

JUNIPER BERRIES

*An evergreen shrub or tree up to 20ft (6m) high, with bluish-green stiff needles. It has small flowers and berries that are green in the first year, black in the second and third.*

### DATAFILE

**AROMATHERAPY/ HOME USE**

**Skin Care:** *Acne, dermatitis, eczema, hair loss, hemorrhoids, oily complexions, wounds.*

**Circulation, Muscles, and Joints:** *Arteriosclerosis, cellulitis, gout, obesity, rheumatism.*

**Immune System:** *Colds, flu.*

**Genitourinary System:** *Amenorrhea, cystitis, dysmenorrhea, leucorrhea.*

**Nervous System:** *Anxiety, tension*

**EXTRACTION**

Essential oil by steam distillation of the berries, needles and wood.

**ACTIONS**

Antirheumatic, antiseptic, antispasmodic, antitoxic, aphrodisiac, astringent, carminative, cicatrizant, depurative, diuretic, emmenagogue, nervine, parasiticide, rubefacient, sedative, stomachic, sudorific, vulnerary.

**COMPATIBILITIES**

Vetiver, sandalwood, cedarwood, mastic, oakmoss, galbanum, elemi, cypress, clary sage, pine, lavender, lavandin, labdanum, fir needle, rosemary, benzoin, balsam tolu, geranium, and citrus oils.

**SAFETY DATA**

*Nonsensitizing, may be slightly irritating, nontoxic. Stimulates the uterine muscle and must not be used during pregnancy. Should not be used by those with kidney disease due to its nephrotoxic effect. Use only juniper berry oil, in moderation*

*JUNIPERUS OXYCEDRUS*

# Cade

FAMILY: CUPRESSACEAE

### Herbal/Folk Tradition

Used in the treatment of cutaneous diseases, such as chronic eczema, parasites, scalp disease, hair loss, etc., especially in France and other European countries. It is also used as an antiseptic wound dressing and for toothache.

FRESH SPRIG

CADE NEEDLES

*A large evergreen shrub up to 13ft (4m) high, with long dark needles and brownish-black berries about the size of hazelnuts.*

## DATAFILE

**AROMATHERAPY/ HOME USE**
Skin Care: *Cuts, blemishes, dandruff, dermatitis, eczema, etc.*

**EXTRACTION**
The crude oil or tar is obtained by destructive distillation from the branches and heartwood (usually in the form of shavings or chips). A rectified oil is produced from the crude by steam or vacuum distillation. An oil is sometimes produced from the berries by steam distillation.

**ACTIONS**
Analgesic, antimicrobial, antipruritic, antiseptic, disinfectant, parasiticide, vermifuge.

**COMPATIBILITIES**
It blends well with thyme, origanum, clove, cassia, tea tree, pine, and medicinal bases.

### SAFETY DATA
*Nontoxic, nonirritant, possible sensitization problems. Use with care, especially when treating inflammatory or allergic skin conditions. Turpentine (terebinth) oil makes a useful alternative, with less possibility of an allergic reaction*

---

*JUNIPERUS SABINA*

# Savine

FAMILY: CUPRESSACEAE

### Herbal/Folk Tradition

It was used at one time as an ointment or dressing for blisters, in order to promote discharge, and for syphilitic warts and other skin problems. It should never be used in pregnancy.

FRESH SPRIG

*A compact evergreen shrub about 3ft (1m) high (much taller around the Mediterranean), which tends to spread horizontally. It has a pale green bark, small, dark green leaves, and purplish-black berries containing three seeds.*

## DATAFILE

**AROMATHERAPY/ HOME USE**
None. Should not be used in therapy, whether internally or externally.

**EXTRACTION**
Essential oil by steam distillation from the twigs and leaves.

**ACTIONS**
Powerful anthelmintic, diuretic, emmenagogue, rubefacient, stimulant, vermifuge.

*Juniperus sabina
Native to North America, middle and southern Europe. The oil is produced mainly in Austria.*

### SAFETY DATA
*Oral toxin. Dermal irritant. Abortifacient. "The oil is banned from sale to the public in many countries due to its toxic effects (nerve poison and blood circulation stimulant)."[18]*

*JUNIPERUS VIRGINIANA*

# Virginian cedarwood

FAMILY: CUPRESSACEAE

## Herbal/Folk Tradition

The Native Americans used it for respiratory infections. Decoctions of leaves, bark, twigs, and fruit were used to treat kidney infections, menstrual delay, gonorrhea, rheumatism, arthritis, skin rashes, venereal warts.

FRESH VIRGINIAN
CEDARWOOD

*A coniferous, slow-growing, evergreen tree up to 108ft (33m) high with a narrow, dense, and pyramidal crown, a reddish heartwood, and brown cones. The trunk diameter can reach over 5ft (1.5m).*

### DATAFILE

**AROMATHERAPY/ HOME USE**

**Skin Care:** *Acne, dandruff, eczema, greasy hair, insect repellent, oily skin, psoriasis.*

**Circulation, Muscles, and Joints:** *Arthritis, rheumatism.*

**Respiratory System:** *Bronchitis, catarrh, congestion, coughs, sinusitis.*

**Genitourinary System:** *Cystitis, leucorrhea.*

**Nervous System:** *Nervous tension and stress-related disorders.*

**EXTRACTION**

Essential oil by steam distillation from the timber waste.

**ACTIONS**

Abortifacient, antiseborrheic, antiseptic (pulmonary, genito-urinary), antispasmodic, astringent, balsamic, diuretic, emmenagogue, expectorant, insecticide, sedative (nervous), stimulant (circulatory).

**COMPATIBILITIES**

It blends well with benzoin, sandalwood, rose, juniper, cypress, vetiver, and patchouli.

**SAFETY DATA**
*See Texas cedarwood, page 93*

---

*LAURUS NOBILIS*

# Bay laurel

FAMILY: LAURACEAE

## Herbal/Folk Tradition

A popular culinary herb throughout Europe. Both leaf and berry were formerly used for a variety of afflictions including hysteria, colic, indigestion, loss of appetite, to promote menstruation, and for fever.

FRESH
BAY LEAF

*An evergreen tree up to 65ft (20m) high with dark green, glossy leaves and black berries; often cultivated as an ornamental shrub.*

### DATAFILE

**AROMATHERAPY/ HOME USE**

**Digestive System:** *Dyspepsia, flatulence, loss of appetite.*

**Genitourinary System:** *Scanty periods.*

**Immune System:** *Colds, flu, tonsillitis, and viral infections.*

**EXTRACTION**

Essential oil by steam distillation from the dried leaf and branchlets. An oil from the berries is produced in small quantities.

**ACTIONS**

Antirheumatic, antiseptic, bactericidal, diaphoretic, digestive, diuretic, emmenagogue, fungicidal, hypotensive, sedative, stomachic.

**COMPATIBILITIES**

It blends well with pine, cypress, juniper, clary sage, rosemary, olibanum, labdanum, lavender, citrus and spice oils.

**SAFETY DATA**
*Relatively nontoxic and nonirritant; can cause dermatitis in some individuals. Use in moderation due to possible narcotic properties attributed to methyl eugenol. Should not be used during pregnancy*

ESSENTIAL OILS

*LAVANDULA ANGUSTIFOLIA*

# True lavender

FAMILY: LAMIACEAE (LABIATAE)

## Herbal/Folk Tradition

Lavender has a well-established tradition as a folk remedy, and its scent is still familiar to almost everyone. It was used to "comfort the stomach" but above all as a cosmetic water, an insect repellent, to scent linen, and as a reviving yet soothing oil. Generally regarded as the most versatile essence therapeutically.

FRESH LAVENDER

*An evergreen woody shrub, up to 3ft (1m) tall, with pale green, narrow, linear leaves and flowers on blunt spikes of a beautiful violet-blue color. The whole plant is highly aromatic.*

## DATAFILE

### AROMATHERAPY/ HOME USE

**Skin Care:** *Abscesses, acne, allergies, athlete's foot, blemishes, all skin types, boils, bruises, burns, dandruff, dermatitis, earache, eczema, inflammations, insect bites and stings, insect repellent, lice, psoriasis, ringworm, scabies, sores, sunburn, wounds.*

**Circulation, Muscles, and Joints:** *Lumbago, muscular aches and pains, rheumatism, sprains.*

**Respiratory System:** *Asthma, bronchitis, catarrh, halitosis, laryngitis, throat infections, whooping cough.*

**Digestive System:** *Abdominal cramps, colic, dyspepsia, flatulence, nausea.*

**Genitourinary System:** *Cystitis, dysmenorrhea, leucorrhea.*

**Immune System:** *Flu.*

**Nervous System:** *Depression, headache, hypertension, insomnia, migraine, nervous tension and stress-related conditions, PMS, sciatica, shock, vertigo.*

### EXTRACTION

Essential oil by steam distillation from the fresh flowering tops. An absolute and concrete are also produced by solvent extraction in smaller quantities.

*Lavandula angustifolia*

### ACTIONS

Analgesic, anticonvulsive, antidepressant, antimicrobial, antirheumatic, antiseptic, antispasmodic, antitoxic, carminative, cholagogue, choleretic, cicatrizant, cordial, cytophylactic, deodorant, diuretic, emmenagogue, hypotensive, insecticide, nervine, parasiticide, rubefacient, sedative, stimulant, sudorific, tonic, vermifuge, vulnerary.

### COMPATIBILITIES

It blends well with most oils, especially citrus and florals; also cedarwood, clove, clary sage, pine, geranium, labdanum, oakmoss, vetiver, and patchouli.

### SAFETY DATA

*Nontoxic, nonirritant, nonsensitizing*

96

*LAVANDULA X INTERMEDIA*

# Lavandin

FAMILY: LAMIACEAE (LABIATAE)

## Herbal/Folk Tradition

Sixty years ago lavandin was still unknown, so it does not have a long history of therapeutic use. Its properties seem to combine those of the true lavender and aspic.

FRESH
LAVANDIN LEAF

*A hybrid plant developed by crossing true lavender (*L. angustifolia*) with spike lavender or aspic (*L. latifolia*). In general, it is a larger plant than true lavender, with woody stems. Its flowers may be blue, or grayish like aspic.*

### DATAFILE

**AROMATHERAPY/ HOME USE**
Similar uses to true lavender, but it is more penetrating and rubefacient with a sharper scent – good for respiratory, circulatory, or muscular conditions.

**EXTRACTION**
Essential oil by steam distillation from the fresh flowering tops; it has a higher yield of oil than either true lavender or apic. (A concrete and absolute are produced by solvent extraction.)

**ACTIONS**
See True lavender, page 96.

**COMPATIBILITIES**
It blends well with clove, bay leaf, cinnamon, citronella, cypress, pine, clary sage, geranium, thyme, patchouli, rosemary, and citrus oils, especially bergamot and lime.

**SAFETY DATA**
*Nontoxic, nonirritant, nonsensitizing*

*LAVANDULA LATIFOLIA*

# Spike lavender

FAMILY: LAMIACEAE (LABIATAE)

## Herbal/Folk Tradition

Culpeper recommends spike lavender for "pains of the head and brain which proceed from cold, apoplexy, falling sickness, the dropsy, or sluggish malady, cramps, convulsions, palsies, and often faintings."[19]

FRESH LEAVES

*An aromatic evergreen subshrub up to 3ft (1m) high with lance-shaped leaves, broader and rougher than those of true lavender. The flower is more compressed and of a dull gray-blue color.*

### DATAFILE

**AROMATHERAPY/ HOME USE**
See True lavender, page 96.

**EXTRACTION**
Essential oil by water or steam distillation from the flowering tops

**ACTIONS**
See True lavender, page 96.

**COMPATIBILITIES**
It blends well with rosemary, sage, lavandin, eucalyptus, rosewood, lavender, petitgrain, pine, cedarwood, oakmoss, patchouli, and spice oils, particularly clove.

*Lavandula latifolia*

**SAFETY DATA**
*Nontoxic, nonirritant (except in concentration), nonsensitizing*

# Lovage

FAMILY: APIACEAE (UMBELLIFERAE)

## Herbal/Folk Tradition

A herb of ancient medical repute, used mainly for digestive complaints, edema, skin problems, menstrual irregularities, and fever. It was also believed to be good for the sight. The leaf stalks used to be blanched and used as a vegetable or in salads. The root is current in the British Herbal Pharmacopoeia as a specific for flatulent dyspepsia and anorexia.

*The oil obtained from the fresh roots is amber or olive-brown, with a rich spicy, warm, rootlike odor.*

FRESH LOVAGE

*A large perennial herb up to 6ft (2m) high with a stout hollow stem and dense ornamental foliage. It has a thick fleshy root and greenish-yellow flowers. The whole plant has a strong aromatic scent.*

---

**DATAFILE**

### AROMATHERAPY/ HOME USE

**Circulation, Muscles, and Joints:**
*Accumulation of toxins, congestion, gout, edema, poor circulation, rheumatism, water retention.*

**Digestive System:**
*Anemia, flatulence, indigestion, spasm.*

**Genitourinary System:**
*Amenorrhea, dysmenorrhea, cystitis.*

### EXTRACTION

Essential oil by steam distillation from the fresh roots and the fresh leaves and stalks of the herb.

### ACTIONS

Antimicrobial, antiseptic, antispasmodic, diaphoretic, digestive, diuretic, carminative, depurative, emmenagogue, expectorant, febrifuge, stimulant (digestive), stomachic.

### COMPATIBILITIES

It blends well with rose, galbanum, costus, opopanax, oakmoss, bay, lavandin, and spice oils.

*Levisticum officinale*

---

**SAFETY DATA**
*Nontoxic, nonirritant, possible sensitization/phototoxic effects. Use with care. Avoid during pregnancy*

*LIQUIDAMBAR ORIENTALIS*

# Levant styrax

FAMILY: HAMAMELIDACEAE

## Herbal/Folk Tradition

In China it is used for coughs, colds, epilepsy, and skin problems, including cuts, wounds, and scabies. It is recommended in the West for catarrh, diphtheria, gonorrhea, leucorrhea, and ringworm.

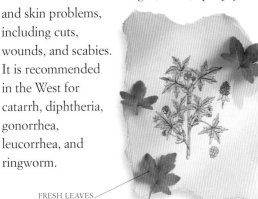

FRESH LEAVES

*A deciduous tree, up to 49ft (15m) high, with a purplish-gray bark, leaves arranged into five three-lobed sections, and white flowers. Styrax is produced by pounding the bark, which induces the sapwood to produce a liquid.*

### DATAFILE

**AROMATHERAPY/ HOME USE**

**Skin Care:** *Cuts, ringworm, scabies, wounds.*

**Respiratory System:** *Bronchitis, catarrh, coughs.*

**Nervous System:** *Anxiety, stress-related conditions.*

**EXTRACTION**

Essential oil by steam distillation from the crude. A resinoid and absolute are also produced by solvent extraction.

**ACTIONS**

Anti-inflammatory, antimicrobial, antiseptic, antitussive, bactericidal, balsamic, expectorant, nervine, stimulant.

**COMPATIBILITIES**

It blends well with ylang ylang, jasmine, mimosa, rose, lavender, carnation, violet, cassie, and spice oils.

### SAFETY DATA
*Nontoxic, nonirritant, possible sensitization in some individuals.*
*Frequently adulterated*

---

*LITSEA CUBEBA*

# Litsea cubeba

FAMILY: LAURACEAE

## Herbal/Folk Tradition

The root and stem are used in Chinese medicine to treat dysmenorrhea, indigestion, lower back pain, chills, headaches, travel sickness, and muscle aches. It may be valuable in treating arrythmia.

FRESH LITSEA CUBEBA

*A small tropical tree with fragrant, lemongrass-scented leaves and flowers. The small fruits are shaped like peppers, from which the name "cubeba" derives.*

### DATAFILE

**AROMATHERAPY/ HOME USE**

**Skin Care:** *Acne, dermatitis, insect repellent, profuse perspiration, .*

**Digestive System:** *Flatulence, indigestion.*

**Immune System:** *Sanitation.*

**Nervous System:** *Arrhythmia, high blood pressure, nervous tension, and stress-related conditions.*

**EXTRACTION**

Essential oil by steam distillation from the fruits.

**ACTIONS**

Antiseptic, deodorant, digestive, disinfectant, insecticidal, sedative, stomachic.

*Litsea cubeba*

### SAFETY DATA
*Nontoxic, nonirritant, possible sensitization in some individuals*

*MATRICARIA RECUTICA*

# German chamomile

FAMILY: ASTERACEAE (COMPOSITAE)

## Herbal/Folk Tradition

This herb has a long-standing medicinal tradition, especially in Europe. An excellent skin care remedy, it has greater anti-inflammatory properties than Roman chamomile.

GERMAN CHAMOMILE SEEDS

*An annual, strongly aromatic herb, up to 24in (60cm) tall, with a hairless, erect, branching stem. It has feathery leaves and simple daisylike white flowers on single stems.*

DATAFILE

### AROMATHERAPY/ HOME USE
See Roman chamomile, page 64.

### EXTRACTION
Essential oil by steam distillation from the flowerheads (up to 1.9 per cent yield). An absolute is also produced in small quantities, which is a deeper blue color and has greater tenacity and fixative properties.

### ACTIONS
Analgesic, antiallergenic, anti-inflammatory, antiphlogistic, antispasmodic, bactericidal, carminative, cicatrizant, cholagogue, digestive, emmenagogue, febrifuge, fungicidal, hepatic, nerve sedative, stimulant of leucocyte production, stomachic, sudorific, vermifuge, vulnerary.

### COMPATIBILITIES
It blends well with geranium, lavender, patchouli, rose, benzoin, neroli, bergamot, marjoram, lemon, ylang ylang, jasmine, clary sage, and labdanum.

**SAFETY DATA**
*Nontoxic, nonirritant, causes dermatitis in some individuals*

---

*MELALEUCA CAJEPUTI*

# Cajeput

FAMILY: MYRTACEAE

FRESH CAJEPUT

## Herbal/Folk Tradition

In the East, it is used locally for colds, headaches, throat infections, toothache, sore muscles, fever rheumatism and various skin diseases. In the West the oil is known for producing a sensation of warmth.

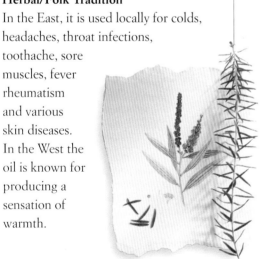

*An evergreen tree up to 98ft (30m) high, with thick pointed leaves and white flowers. The flexible trunk has a whitish spongy bark that flakes off easily.*

DATAFILE

### AROMATHERAPY/ HOME USE
Skin Care: *Blemishes, insect bites, oily skin.*
Circulation, Muscles, and Joints: *Arthritis, muscular aches and pains, rheumatism.*
Respiratory System: *Asthma, bronchitis, catarrh, coughs, sinusitis, sore throat.*
Genitourinary System: *Cystitis, urethritis, urinary infection.*
Immune System:
*Colds, flu, viral infections.*

### EXTRACTION
Essential oil by steam distillation from the fresh leaves and twigs.

### ACTIONS
Mildly analgesic, antimicrobial, antineuralgic, antispasmodic, antiseptic (pulmonary, urinary, intestinal), anthelmintic, diaphoretic, carminative, expectorant, febrifuge, insecticide, sudorific, tonic.

**SAFETY DATA**
*Nontoxic, nonsensitizing, may irritate the skin in high concentration*

*MELALEUCA ALTERNIFOLIA*

# Tea tree

FAMILY: MYRTACEAE

## Herbal/Folk Tradition

The name derives from its local usage as a type of herbal tea, prepared from the leaves. Our present  knowledge of tea tree is based on a very long history of use by the aboriginal people of Australia. It has been extensively researched by scientific methods with the following results: "1. This oil is unusual in that it is active against all three varieties of infectious organisms: bacteria, fungi, and viruses. 2. It is a very powerful immuno-stimulant, so when the body is threatened by any of these organisms ti-tree increases its ability to respond."[20]

*A small tree or shrub (smallest of the tea tree family), with needle-like leaves similar to cypress, with heads of sessile yellow or purplish flowers.*

DRIED TEA
TREE FLOWERS

**DATAFILE**

### AROMATHERAPY/HOME USE

**Skin Care:** *Abscess, acne, athlete's foot, blemishes, blisters, burns, cold sores, dandruff, herpes, insect bites, oily skin, plantar warts (verrucae), rashes (diaper rash), warts, wounds (infected).*
**Respiratory System:** *Asthma, bronchitis, catarrh, coughs, sinusitis, tuberculosis, whooping cough.*
**Genitourinary System:** *Thrush, vaginitis, cystitis, pruritis.*
**Immune System:** *Colds, fever, flu, infectious illnesses such as chickenpox.*

### EXTRACTION

Essential oil by distillation (steam) from leaves and twigs.

### ACTIONS

Anti-infectious, anti-inflammatory, antiseptic, antiviral, bactericidal, balsamic, cicatrizant, diaphoretic, expectorant, fungicidal, immunostimulant, parasiticide, vulnerary.

### COMPATIBILITIES

Lavandin, lavender, clary sage, rosemary, oakmoss, pine, cananga, geranium, marjoram, and spice oils,

*Melaleuca alternifolia*

**SAFETY DATA**
*Nontoxic, nonirritant, possible sensitization in some individuals*

*MELALEUCA VIRIDIFLORA*

# Niaouli

FAMILY: MYRTACEAE

### Herbal/Folk Tradition

Native to Australia, New Caledonia, and the French Pacific Islands, it is used locally for a wide variety of ailments, such as aches and pains, respiratory conditions, cuts, and infections; it is also used to purify water.

NIAOULI NEEDLES

*An evergreen tree with a flexible trunk and spongy bark, pointed linear leaves, and spikes of sessile yellowish flowers. The leaves have a strong aromatic scent when crushed.*

DATAFILE

**AROMATHERAPY/ HOME USE**
**Skin Care:** *Acne, blemishes, boils, burns, cuts, insect bites, oily skin, ulcers, wounds.*
**Circulation, Muscles, and Joints:** *Muscular aches and pains, poor circulation, rheumatism.*
**Respiratory System:** *Asthma, bronchitis, catarrhal conditions, coughs, sinusitis, sore throat, whooping cough.*
**Genitourinary System:** *Cystitis, urinary infection.*
**Immune System:** *Colds, fever, flu.*

**EXTRACTION**
Essential oil by steam distillation from the leaves and young twigs. (Usually rectified to remove irritant aldehydes.)

**ACTIONS**
Analgesic, anthelmintic, anticatarrhal, antirheumatic, antiseptic, antispasmodic, bactericidal, balsamic, cicatrizant, diaphoretic, expectorant, regulator, stimulant, vermifuge.

**SAFETY DATA**
*Nontoxic, nonirritant, nonsensitizing. Often subject to adulteration*

---

*MELILOTUS OFFICINALIS*

# Melilotus

FAMILY: FABACEAE (LEGUMINOSAE)

### Herbal/Folk Tradition

The leaves and shoots are used in continental Europe for conditions that include sleeplessness, thrombosis, tension, varicose veins, intestinal disorders, headache, and earache.

DRIED MELILOTUS

*A bushy perennial herb up to 3ft (1m) high, with smooth erect stems, trifoliate oval leaves, and small sweet-scented white or yellow flowers – their scent is stronger on drying.*

DATAFILE

**AROMATHERAPY/ HOME USE**
None.

**EXTRACTION**
A concrete (usually called a resinoid or oleoresin) by solvent extraction from the dry flowers

**ACTIONS**
Anti-inflammatory, antirheumatic, antispasmodic, astringent, emollient, expectorant, digestive, insecticidal (against moth), sedative.

*Melilotus officinalis Native to Europe and Asia Minor. The oleoresin is used in high-quality perfumery work.*

**SAFETY DATA**
*In 1953 in some countries, including the United States, coumarin was banned from use in flavorings due to toxicity levels. Some coumarins are also known to be phototoxic.*

*MELISSA OFFICINALIS*

# Lemon balm

FAMILY: LAMIACEAE (LABIATAE)

## Herbal/Folk Tradition

One of the earliest known medicinal herbs, associated with nervous disorders, the heart, and the emotions. It is generally used for respiratory and digestive complaints of nervous origin such as asthma, indigestion, and flatulence.

FRESH LEAVES

*A sweet-scented herb about 24in (60cm) high, soft and bushy, with bright green serrated leaves, square stems, and tiny white or pink flowers.*

### DATAFILE

**AROMATHERAPY/HOME USE**

**Skin Care:** *Allergies, insect bites and repellent. Low concentrations can be used to treat eczema and other skin problems.*

**Respiratory System:** *Asthma, bronchitis, chronic coughs.*

**Digestive System:** *Colic, indigestion, nausea.*

**Genitourinary System:** *Menstrual problems.*

**Nervous System:** *Anxiety, depression, hypertension, insomnia, migraine, nervous tension, shock, and vertigo.*

**EXTRACTION**

Essential oil by steam distillation from leaves and flowering tops.

**ACTIONS**

Antidepressant, antihistaminic, antispasmodic, bactericidal, carminative, cordial, diaphoretic, emmenagogue, febrifuge, hypertensive, nervine, sedative, stomachic, sudorific, tonic, uterine, vermifuge.

**COMPATIBILITIES**

It blends well with lavender, geranium, floral and citrus oils.

#### SAFETY DATA

*Nontoxic. Possible sensitization and dermal irritation: use in low dilutions only. One of the most frequently adulterated oils. Most commercial so-called melissa contains some or all of the following: lemon, lemongrass, or citronella*

---

*MENTHA ARVENSIS*

# Cornmint

FAMILY: LAMIACEAE (LABIATAE)

## Herbal/Folk Tradition

Used therapeutically in many of the same ways as peppermint. In the East it is used to treat rheumatic pain, neuralgia, toothache, laryngitis, indigestion, colds, and bronchitis.

FRESH CORNMINT LEAVES

*A somewhat fragile herb with leafy stems up to 24in (60cm) high, lance-shaped leaves and lilac-colored flowers borne in clustered whorls in the axils of the upper leaves.*

### DATAFILE

**AROMATHERAPY/HOME USE**

Not compatible with homeopathic treatment. Use Peppermint, see page 104, in preference, since it is not fractionated like the commercial cornmint oil and has a more refined fragrance.

**EXTRACTION**

Essential oil by steam distillation from the flowering herb. The oil is usually dementholized since it contains so much menthol that it is otherwise solid at room temperature.

*Mentha arvensis*
*Native to Europe, Japan, and China, and naturalized in North America.*

**ACTIONS**

Anesthetic, antimicrobial, antiseptic, antispasmodic, carminative, cytotoxic, digestive, expectorant, stimulant, stomachic.

#### SAFETY DATA

*Nontoxic, nonirritant (except in concentration); may cause sensitization in some individuals. Menthol is a dermal irritant.*

*MENTHA PIPERITA*

# Peppermint

FAMILY: LAMIACEAE (LABIATAE)

FRESH PEPPERMINT LEAVES

## Herbal/Folk Tradition

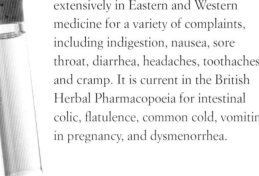

Mints have been cultivated since ancient times in China and Japan. In Egypt evidence of a type of peppermint has been found in tombs dating from 1000 BCE. It has been used extensively in Eastern and Western medicine for a variety of complaints, including indigestion, nausea, sore throat, diarrhea, headaches, toothaches, and cramp. It is current in the British Herbal Pharmacopoeia for intestinal colic, flatulence, common cold, vomiting in pregnancy, and dysmenorrhea.

*A perennial herb up to 3ft (1m) high with underground runners by which it is easily propagated. The "white" peppermint has green stems and leaves; the "black" peppermint has dark green serrated leaves, purplish stems, and reddish-violet flowers.*

---

### DATAFILE

#### AROMATHERAPY/HOME USE
Not compatible with homeopathic treatment.
**Skin Care:** *Acne, dermatitis, ringworm, scabies, toothache.*
**Circulation, Muscles, and Joints:** *Neuralgia, muscular pain, palpitations.*
**Respiratory System:** *Asthma, bronchitis, halitosis, sinusitis, spasmodic cough – "When inhaled (in steam) it checks catarrh temporarily, and will provide relief from head colds and bronchitis: its antispasmodic action combines well with this to make it a most useful inhalation in asthma."[21]*

**Digestive System:** *Colic, cramp, dyspepsia, flatulence, nausea.*
**Immune System:** *Colds, flu, fevers.*
**Nervous System:** *Fainting, headache, mental fatigue, migraine, nervous stress, vertigo.*

#### EXTRACTION
Essential oil by steam distillation from the flowering herb (approx. 3–4 per cent yield).

*Mentha piperita*

#### ACTIONS
Analgesic, anti-inflammatory, antimicrobial, antiphlogistic, antipruritic, antiseptic, antispasmodic, antiviral, astringent, carminative, cephalic, cholagogue, cordial, emmenagogue, expectorant, febrifuge, hepatic, nervine, stomachic, sudorific, vasoconstrictor, vermifuge.

#### COMPATIBILITIES
It blends well with benzoin, rosemary, lavender, marjoram, lemon, eucalyptus, and other mints.

---

### SAFETY DATA
*Nontoxic, nonirritant (except in concentration), possible sensitization due to menthol. Use in moderation*

*MENTHA PULEGIUM*

# Pennyroyal

FAMILY: LAMIACEAE (LABIATAE)

### Herbal/Folk Tradition
A herbal remedy of ancient repute, used for a wide variety of ailments. It was believed to purify the blood and be able to communicate its purifying qualities to water.

DRIED PENNYROYAL

*A perennial herb up to 20in (50cm) tall with smooth roundish stalks, small pale purple flowers, and aromatic, gray-green oval leaves. It has a fibrous creeping root.*

**AROMATHERAPY/HOME USE**
None. It should not be used in aromatherapy, either internally or externally.

**EXTRACTION**
Essential oil by steam distillation from the fresh or slightly dried herb.

**ACTIONS**
Antiseptic, antispasmodic, diaphoretic, carminative, digestive, emmenagogue, insect repellent, refrigerant, stimulant.

*Mentha pulegium*

**COMPATIBILITIES**
It blends well with geranium, rosemary, lavandin, sage, and citronella.

**SAFETY DATA**
Oral toxin. Abortifacient (due to pulegone content). Ingestion of large doses has resulted in death

---

*MENTHA SPICATA*

# Spearmint

FAMILY: LAMIACEAE (LABIATAE)

### Herbal/Folk Tradition
Valued all over the world as a culinary herb. The ancient Greeks used it to scent their bathwater. The distilled water is used to relieve hiccups, colic, nausea, indigestion, and flatulence.

FRESH SPEARMINT

*A hardy branched perennial herb with bright green, lance-shaped, sharply serrated leaves, quickly spreading underground runners, and pink or lilac-colored flowers in slender cylindrical spikes.*

**DATAFILE**

**AROMATHERAPY/HOME USE**
Not compatible with homeopathic treatment. Less powerful than peppermint oil, it is useful for the treatment of children's maladies.
**Skin Care:** *Acne, dermatitis, congested skin.*
**Respiratory System:** *Asthma, bronchitis, catarrhal conditions, sinusitis.*
**Digestive System:** *Colic, dyspepsia, flatulence, hepatobiliary disorders, nausea.*
**Immune System:** *Colds, fevers.*
**Nervous System:** *Fatigue, headache, migraine, nervous strain, neurasthenia, stress.*

**EXTRACTION**
Essential oil by steam distillation from the flowering tops.

**ACTIONS**
Anesthetic (local), antiseptic, antispasmodic, astringent, carminative, cephalic, cholagogue, decongestant, digestive, diuretic, expectorant, febrifuge, hepatic, nervine, stimulant, stomachic, tonic.

**COMPATIBILITIES**
It blends well with lavender, lavandin, jasmine, eucalyptus, basil, and rosemary and is often used in combination with peppermint.

**SAFETY DATA**
Nontoxic, nonirritant, nonsensitizing

*MYRISTICA FRAGRANS*

# Nutmeg

FAMILY: MYRISTICACEAE

### Herbal/Folk Tradition

Nutmeg and mace are widely used as domestic spices and have been used for centuries as a remedy for kidney and digestive problems. Grated nutmeg with lard is used for piles. A fixed oil of nutmeg is also used in soap and candle-making.

DRIED NUTMEG SEED

*Evergreen tree up to 65ft (20m) high with a grayish-brown smooth bark, dense foliage, and small dull-yellow flowers.*

**DATAFILE**

**AROMATHERAPY/ HOME USE**
Use in moderation, and with care in pregnancy.
**Circulation, Muscles, and Joints**: *Arthritis, gout, muscular aches and pains, poor circulation, rheumatism.*
**Digestive System**: *Flatulence, indigestion, nausea.*
**Immune System**: *Bacterial infection.*
**Nervous System**: *Frigidity, impotence, neuralgia, fatigue.*

**EXTRACTION**
Essential oil by steam (or water) distillation from the dried seed, or the husk (mace). Oleoresin by solvent extraction from mace.

**ACTIONS**
Analgesic, antiemetic, antioxidant, antirheumatic, antiseptic, antispasmodic, aphrodisiac, carminative, digestive, emmenagogue, gastric secretory stimulant, larvicidal, orexigenic, prostaglandin inhibitor, stimulant.

**COMPATIBILITIES**
Oakmoss, lavandin, bay leaf, Peru balsam, orange, geranium, clary sage, rosemary, lime, petitgrain, mandarin, spice oils.

**SAFETY DATA**
*Nutmeg and mace are generally nontoxic, nonirritant and nonsensitizing. However, used in large doses they show signs of toxicity such as nausea, stupor, and tachycardia, believed to be due to the myristicin content*

*MYROCARPUS FASTIGIATUS*

# Cabreuva

FAMILY: FABACEAE (LEGUMINOSAE)

### Herbal/Folk Tradition

The wood is highly appreciated for carving and furniture-making. It is used locally to heal wounds, ulcers, and to obviate scars. It was listed in old European pharmacopoeias for its antiseptic qualities.

CABREUVA WOOD CHIPPINGS

*A graceful, tall tropical tree, 39–49ft (12–15m) high, with a very hard wood, extremely resistant to moisture and mold growth. It yields a balsam when the trunk is damaged, like many other South American trees.*

**DATAFILE**

**AROMATHERAPY/ HOME USE**
**Skin Care**: *Cuts, scars, wounds.*
**Respiratory System:**
*Chills, coughs.*
**Immune System**: *Colds.*

**EXTRACTION**
Essential oil by steam distillation from wood chippings.

**ACTIONS**
Antiseptic, balsamic, cicatrizant.

**COMPATIBILITIES**
It blends well with rose, cassie, mimosa, cedarwood, and rich woody and oriental bases.

**SAFETY DATA**
*Nontoxic, nonirritant, nonsensitizing*

*MYROXYLON BALSAMUM VAR. BALSAMUM*

# Tolu balsam

FAMILY: FABACEAE (LEGUMINOSAE)

### Herbal/Folk Tradition

It works primarily on the respiratory mucous membranes and is good for non-inflammatory chest complaints, chronic catarrh, croup, and laryngitis. It is used in cough syrups and lozenges.

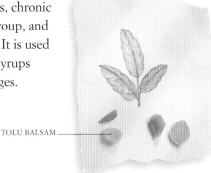

TOLU BALSAM

*A tall tropical tree, similar in appearance to the Peru balsam tree. The balsam is obtained by making V-shaped incisions into the bark and sap wood, often after the trunk has been beaten and scorched. It is a "true" balsam.*

### DATAFILE

**AROMATHERAPY/ HOME USE**

Skin Care: *Dry, chapped and cracked skin, eczema, rashes, scabies, sores, wounds.*

Respiratory System: *Bronchitis, catarrh, coughs, croup, laryngitis. "Use as an inhalant by putting about a teaspoon into a steam bath."[22]*

**EXTRACTION**

The crude balsam is collected from the trees. It appears first in liquid form, then solidifies into a brittle mass. An essential oil is obtained from the crude by steam or dry distillation.

**ACTIONS**

Antitussive, antiseptic, balsamic, expectorant, stimulant.

**COMPATIBILITIES**

It blends well with mimosa, ylang ylang, sandalwood, labdanum, orange blossom, patchouli, cedarwood, and oriental, spicy, and floral bases.

**SAFETY DATA**

*Available information indicates it to be nontoxic, nonirritant, possible sensitization; see Peru balsam (below)*

---

*MYROXYLON BALSAMUM VAR. PEREIRAE*

# Peru balsam

FAMILY: FABACEAE (LEGUMINOSAE)

### Herbal/Folk Tradition

It stimulates the heart, increases blood pressure, and lessens mucous secretions, and is useful for respiratory disorders such as asthma, chronic coughs, and bronchitis.

PERU BALSAM LEAVES

*A large tropical tree up to 82ft (25m) high, with a straight smooth trunk, beautiful foliage, and fragrant flowers. Every part of the tree contains a resinous juice. Balsam is obtained from the exposed wood after the bark has been stripped.*

### DATAFILE

**AROMATHERAPY/ HOME USE**

The balsam (not the oil) is a common contact allergen, which may cause dermatitis. Those who have this sensitivity may also react to benzoin resinoid ("cross-sensitization").

Skin Care: *Dry and chapped skin, eczema, rashes, sores, and wounds.*

Circulation, Muscles, and Joints: *Low blood pressure, rheumatism.*

Respiratory System: *Asthma, bronchitis, coughs.*

Immune System: *Colds.*

Nervous System: *Nervous tension, stress.*

**EXTRACTION**

Resin-free essential oil is produced from crude balsam by high vacuum dry distillation. (A wood oil, which is considered of inferior quality, is produced by steam distillation from wood chippings.)

**ACTIONS**

Anti-inflammatory, antiseptic, balsamic, expectorant, parasiticide, stimulant; promotes the growth of epithelial cells.

**COMPATIBILITIES**

It blends well with ylang ylang, patchouli, petitgrain, sandalwood, rose, spices, and floral and oriental bases.

**SAFETY DATA**

*Nontoxic, nonirritant*

# Myrtle

FAMILY: MYRTACEAE

## Herbal/Folk Tradition

The leaves and berries were traditionally thought to be good for diarrhea, dysentery, and catarrh. The leaves and flowers were a major ingredient of "angel's water", a sixteenth-century skin-care lotion.

FRESH MYRTLE

*A large, fragrant bush or small tree with many tough but slender branches, a brownish-red bark, and small pointed leaves. It has white flowers followed by small black berries.*

### DATAFILE

**AROMATHERAPY/ HOME USE**

**Skin Care:** *Acne, hemorrhoids, oily skin, open pores.*

**Respiratory System:** *Asthma, bronchitis, catarrhal conditions, chronic coughs, tuberculosis – it is a suitable oil to use for children's coughs and chest complaints.*

**Immune System:** *Colds, flu, infectious disease.*

**EXTRACTION**

Essential oil by steam distillation from the leaves and twigs, and sometimes the flowers.

*Myrtus communis*

**ACTIONS**

Anticatarrhal, antiseptic (urinary, pulmonary), astringent, balsamic, bactericidal, expectorant, regulator, slightly sedative.

**COMPATIBILITIES**

Bergamot, lavandin, lavender, clary sage, rosemary, hyssop, bay leaf, lime, laurel, ginger, and spice oils.

**SAFETY DATA**
*Nontoxic, nonirritant, nonsensitizing*

---

# Narcissus

FAMILY: AMARYLLIDACEAE

## Herbal/Folk Tradition

The name derives from its narcotic properties; the Greek *narkao* means "to be numb". In France the flowers were used at one time for their antispasmodic properties, said to be useful in hysteria and epilepsy.

NARCISSUS BULB

*A familiar garden flower up to 20in (50cm) high, with long sword-shaped leaves and very fragrant white flowers, having a short yellow trumpet and crisped red edge.*

### DATAFILE

**AROMATHERAPY/ HOME USE**

**Perfume.** The bulbs of N. poeticus are more dangerous than those of the daffodil, since they have powerful emetic and irritant qualities. If the flowers are present in any quantity in a closed room, they will produce headache and even vomiting in some people.

**EXTRACTION**

A concrete and absolute by solvent extraction from the flowers.

**ACTIONS**

Antispasmodic, aphrodisiac, emetic, narcotic, sedative.

**COMPATIBILITIES**

It blends well with clove bud, jasmine, neroli, ylang ylang, rose, mimosa, sandalwood, oriental and floral fragrances.

**SAFETY DATA**
*All members of the Amaryllidaceae family, especially the bulbs, have a profound effect on the nervous system, causing paralysis and even, in some cases, death*

*NARDOSTACHYS JATAMANSI*

# Spikenard

FAMILY: VALERIANANCEAE

## Herbal/Folk Tradition

Spikenard is one of the early aromatics used by the ancient Egyptians and is mentioned in the *Song of Solomon* in the Bible.
The herb was considered good for nausea, flatulent indigestion, menstrual problems, inflammations, and conjunctivitis.

DRIED SPIKENARD ROOT

*A tender aromatic herb with a pungent rhizome root.*

**AROMATHERAPY/ HOME USE**
Skin Care: *Allergies, inflammation, mature skin (rejuvenating), rashes, etc.*
Nervous System: *Insomnia, nervous indigestion, migraine, stress, and tension.*

**EXTRACTION**
Essential oil by steam distillation from the dried and crushed rhizome and roots.

**ACTIONS**
Anti-inflammatory, antipyretic, bactericidal, deodorant, fungicidal, laxative, sedative, tonic.

**COMPATIBILITIES**
It blends well with labdanum, lavender, oakmoss, patchouli, pine needle, vetiver, and spice oils.

**SAFETY DATA**
Probably similar to Valerian, see page 134, i.e. nontoxic, nonirritant, nonsensitizing

---

*OCIMUM BASILICUM*

# Exotic basil

FAMILY: LAMIACEAE (LABIATAE)

## Herbal/Folk Tradition

A popular culinary herb, especially in Italy and France. In the West it is considered a cooling herb and is used for rheumatic pain, irritable skin conditions, and for those of a nervous disposition. It is also widely used in Far Eastern medicine.

LEAVES

FRESH BASIL FLOWERS

*Botanically classified as identical with French basil, though it is a larger plant with a harsher odor and different constituents.*

**DATAFILE**

**AROMATHERAPY/ HOME USE**
None.
Exotic basil is produced mainly in the Comoran Islands. It has a high methyl chavicol content, which is sufficient reason to discard it for therapeutic usage in favor of the French type.

**EXTRACTION**
Essential oil by steam distillation from the leaves and flowering tops.

**ACTIONS**
Antidepressant, antiseptic, antispasmodic, carminative,

*Ocimum basilicum*

cephalic, digestive, emmenagogue, expectorant, febrifuge, galactagogue, nervine, prophlyactic, restorative, stimulant of adrenal cortex, stomachic, tonic.

**SAFETY DATA**
Methyl chavicol is moderately toxic, irritating to the skin, and may be carcinogenic. Basil should be avoided during pregnancy

*OCIMUM BASILICUM*

# French basil

FAMILY: LAMIACEAE (LABIATAE)

## Herbal/Folk Tradition
See Exotic basil, page 109.

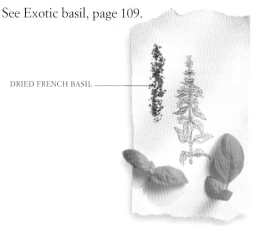

DRIED FRENCH BASIL

*A tender, aromatic annual herb, with very dark green, ovate leaves, grayish-green beneath, an erect square stem up to 24in (60cm) high, bearing whorls of two-lipped greenish or pinky-white flowers.*

### DATAFILE

**AROMATHERAPY/ HOME USE**

**Skin Care:** *Insect bites (mosquito, wasp), insect repellent.*

**Circulation, Muscles, and Joints:** *Gout, muscular aches and pains, rheumatism.*

**Respiratory System:** *Bronchitis, coughs, earache, sinusitis.*

**Digestive System:** *Dyspepsia, flatulence, nausea.*

**Genitourinary System**: *Cramps, scanty periods.*

**Immune System:** *Colds, fever, flu, infectious disease.*

**Nervous System:** *Anxiety, depression, fatigue, insomnia, migraine, nervous tension.*

**EXTRACTION**
Essential oil by steam distillation from the flowering herb.

**ACTIONS**
See Exotic basil, page 109.

**COMPATIBILITIES**
It blends well with bergamot, clary sage, lime, opopanax, oakmoss, citronella, geranium, hyssop, and other "green" notes.

**SAFETY DATA**
*Relatively nontoxic, nonirritant, possible sensitization in some individuals. Avoid during pregnancy*

---

*ORIGANUM MARJORANA*

# Sweet marjoram

FAMILY: LAMIACEAE (LABIATAE)

## Herbal/Folk Tradition
A traditional culinary herb and folk remedy. It is a versatile herb, and is fortifying, soothing, and warming; it aids digestive and menstrual problems, and nervous and respiratory complaints.

DRIED SWEET MARJORAM

*A tender bushy perennial plant (cultivated as an annual in colder climates), up to 24in (60cm) high with a hairy stem, dark green oval leaves, and small grayish-white flowers in clusters or "knots". The whole plant is strongly aromatic.*

### DATAFILE

**AROMATHERAPY/ HOME USE**

**Skin Care:** *Chilblains, bruises, ticks.*

**Circulation, Muscles, and Joints:** *Arthritis, lumbago, muscular aches, rheumatism, sprains.*

**Respiratory System:** *Asthma, bronchitis, coughs.*

**Digestive System:** *Flatulence colic, constipation, dyspepsia, .*

**Genitourinary System:** *Amenorrhea, dysmenorrhea, leucorrhea, PMS.*

**Immune System:** *Colds.*

**Nervous System:** *Headache, hypertension, insomnia, migraine, tension, and stress.*

**EXTRACTION**
Essential oil by steam distillation of the dried flowering herb.

**ACTIONS**
Analgesic, anaphrodisiac, antioxidant, antiseptic, anti-spasmodic, antiviral, bactericidal, carminative, cephalic, cordial, diaphoretic, digestive, diuretic, emmenagogue, expectorant, fungicidal, hypotensive, laxative, nervine, sedative, stomachic, tonic, vasodilator, vulnerary.

**COMPATIBILITIES**
Lavender, rosemary, bergamot, chamomile, cypress, cedarwood, tea tree, and eucalyptus.

**SAFETY DATA**
*Nontoxic, nonirritant, nonsensitizing. Not to be used during pregnancy*

*ORIGANUM VULGARE*

# Common oregano

FAMILY: LAMIACEAE (LABIATAE)

### Herbal/Folk Tradition

A herb of very ancient medical repute. Traditionally used for digestive upsets, respiratory problems (asthma, bronchitis, coughs, etc.), colds, and flu, as well as for inflammations of the mouth and throat.

DRIED HERB

*A hardy, bushy, perennial herb up to 35in (90cm) high with an erect hairy stem, dark green ovate leaves, and pinky-purple flowers. A common garden plant with a strong aroma when the leaves are bruised.*

### DATAFILE

**AROMATHERAPY/ HOME USE**
None. Do not use on the skin.

**EXTRACTION**
Essential oil by steam distillation from the dried flowering herb.

**ACTIONS**
Analgesic, anthelmintic, anti-rheumatic, antiseptic, anti-spasmodic, antitoxic, antiviral, bactericidal, carminative, choleretic, cytoplactic, diaphoretic, diuretic, emmenagogue, expectorant, febrifuge, fungicidal, parasiticide, rubefacient, stimulant, tonic.

*Origanum vulgare*

**COMPATIBILITIES**
It blends well with lavandin, oakmoss, pine, spike lavender, citronella, rosemary, camphor, and cedarwood.

**SAFETY DATA**
*Dermal toxin, skin irritant, mucous membrane irritant. Avoid during pregnancy*

---

*ORMENIS MULTICAULIS*

# Maroc chamomile

FAMILY: ASTERACEAE (COMPOSITAE)

### Herbal/Folk Tradition

This is one of the more recent oils to appear on the market, and as such it does not have a long history of usage. The oil is distinctly different from the German or the Roman chamomile oils, and is not a replacement.

DRIED MAROC CHAMOMILE

*A handsome plant, 35–49in (90–125cm) high, with very hairy leaves and tubular yellow flowers, surrounded by white ligulets.*

### DATAFILE

**AROMATHERAPY/ HOME USE**
Little is known about its therapeutic history and usage. It has been recommended for sensitive skin, colic, colitis, headache, insomnia, irritability, migraine, amenorrhea, menopause, liver and spleen congestion.

**EXTRACTION**
Essential oil by steam distillation from the flowering tops.

**ACTIONS**
Antispasmodic, cholagogue, emmenagogue, hepatic, sedative.

**COMPATIBILITIES**
It blends well with cypress, lavender, lavandin, vetiver, cedarwood, oakmoss, labdanum, olibanum, and artemisia oils.

**SAFETY DATA**
*Generally nontoxic and nonirritant – more specific safety data is unavailable at present*

*PELARGONIUM GRAVEOLENS*

# Geranium

FAMILY: GERANIACEAE

### Herbal/Folk Tradition

The British plant herb *Geranium robertanium*
and the American *G. maculatum*
are the most widely
used types in
herbal medicine
today. They are
used for
conditions
such as
dysentery and
hemorrhoids.

FRESH LEAVES

*A perennial hairy shrub up to 3ft (1m) high with pointed
leaves, serrated at the edges, and small pink flowers. The
whole plant is aromatic.*

**DATAFILE**

**AROMATHERAPY/ HOME USE**
Skin Care: *Acne, bruises, burns,
congested skin, cuts, dermatitis,
eczema, hemorrhoids, lice, mature
skin, mosquito repellent, oily skin,
ringworm, ulcers, wounds.*
Circulation, Muscles, and Joints:
*Cellulitis, breast engorgement,
edema, poor circulation.*
Respiratory System: *Sore throat,
tonsillitis.*
Genitourinary and Endocrine
Systems: *Adrenocortical glands
and menopausal problems, PMS.*
Nervous System: *Tension,
neuralgia, and stress.*

**EXTRACTION**
Essential oil by steam distillation
from leaves, stalks, and flowers.

**ACTIONS**
Antidepressant, antihemorrhagic,
antiflammatory, antiseptic,
astringent, cicatrizant,
deodorant, diuretic, fungicidal,
hemostatic, stimulant (adrenal
cortex), styptic, tonic,
vermifuge, vulnerary.

**COMPATIBILITIES**
Lavender, patchouli, clove, rose,
orange blossom, sandalwood,
jasmine, juniper, bergamot, and
other citrus oils.

**SAFETY DATA**
*Nontoxic, nonirritant, generally nonsensitizing; possibly contact dermatitis
in hypersensitive individuals, especially with the Bourbon type*

*PETROSELINUM SATIVUM*

# Parsley

FAMILY: APIACEAE (UMBELLIFERAE)

### Herbal/Folk Tradition

Used extensively as a culinary herb, it is a very
nutritious plant, high in vitamins A
and C. The herb
and seed are used
medicinally,
principally for
kidney and
bladder
problems.

FRESH PARSLEY

*A biennial or short-lived perennial herb up to 28in (70cm)
high with crinkly bright green foliage, small greenish-yellow
flowers, and producing small brown seeds.*

**DATAFILE**

**AROMATHERAPY/ HOME USE**
Circulation, Muscles, and Joints:
*Accumulation of toxins, arthritis,
broken blood vessels, cellulites,
rheumatism, sciatica.*
Digestive System: *Colic,
flatulence, indigestion, hemorrhoids.*
Genitourinary System:
*Amenorrhea, dysmenorrhea, to aid
labor, cystitis, urinary infection.*

**EXTRACTION**
Essential oil by steam distillation
from the seed and the herb. An
essential oil is occasionally
extracted from the roots, and

an oleoresin is also produced by
solvent extraction from the
seeds.

**ACTIONS**
Antimicrobial, antirheumatic,
antiseptic, astringent,
carminative, diuretic, depurative,
emmenagogue, febrifuge,
hypotensive, laxative, stimulant
(mild), stomachic, tonic (uterine).

**COMPATIBILITIES**
It blends well with rose, orange
blossom, cananga, tea tree,
oakmoss, clary sage, and spice
oils.

**SAFETY DATA**
*Both oils are moderately toxic and irritant, otherwise nonsensitizing.
Use in moderation. Avoid during pregnancy*

*PEUMUS BOLDUS*

# Boldo leaf

FAMILY: MONIMIACEAE

### Herbal/Folk Tradition

In South America it has long been recognized as a valuable cure for gonorrhea. In Western herbalism, the dried leaves are used for genitourinary inflammation, gallstones, liver or gall bladder pain, cystitis, and rheumatism.

DRIED BOLDO LEAF

*An evergreen shrub or small tree up to 20ft (6m) high, with slender branches, sessile coarse leaves, and bearing yellowish-green fruit; dried the leaves turn a deep reddish-brown color. The whole plant is aromatic.*

**DATAFILE**

**AROMATHERAPY/ HOME USE**

None. The oil has powerful therapeutic effects and should be considered harmful to the human organism even in very small doses It should not be used in therapy, either internally or externally.

**EXTRACTION**

Essential oil by steam distillation of the leaves.

**ACTIONS**

Antiseptic, cholagogue, diaphoretic, diuretic, hepatic, sedative, tonic, urinary demulcent.

*Peumus boldus*
*Native to Chile, naturalized in the Mediterranean region. Some essential oil is produced in Nepal and Vietnam.*

**SAFETY DATA**
Extremely toxic

*PILOCARPUS JABORANDI*

# Jaborandi

FAMILY: RUTACEAE

### Herbal/Folk Tradition

Jaborandi induces salivation and most gland secretions; it was also used at one time to promote hair growth. It is considered useful in psoriasis, prurigo, deafness, chronic catarrh, tonsillitis, and particularly dropsy.

DRIED JABORANDI FLOWERS

*A woody shrub up to 6ft (2m) high with a smooth, grayish bark, large brownish-green leathery leaves containing big oil glands, and reddish-purple flowers.*

**DATAFILE**

**AROMATHERAPY/ HOME USE**

None. Some hypodermic solutions are prepared from pilocarpine, the main active constituent. It is little used in perfumery or flavor work, because of its extreme toxicity.

**EXTRACTION**

Essential oil by steam distillation from the dried leaflets.

**ACTIONS**

Antiseptic, diaphoretic, emmenagogue, galactagogue, stimulant (nerve).

**SAFETY DATA**
Oral toxin, skin irritant, abortifacient

*PIMENTA DIOICA*

# Allspice

FAMILY: MYRTACEAE

### Herbal/Folk Tradition

Used for flatulent indigestion and externally for neuralgic or rheumatic pain. Pimento water helps prevent griping pains and is used as a vehicle for medicines that ease dyspepsia and constipation.

FRESH
ALLSPICE LEAF

*An evergreen tree up to 33ft (10m) high. It produces fruit in its third year. Each fruit contains two kidney-shaped green seeds, which turn glossy black when ripe.*

## DATAFILE

**AROMATHERAPY/ HOME USE**

**Circulation, Muscles, and Joints:** *Arthritis, fatigue, muscle cramp, rheumatism, stiffness, etc. Can be used in tiny amounts in a massage oil for chest infections, severe muscle spasm, or extreme cold.*
**Respiratory System:** *Chills, congested coughs, bronchitis.*
**Digestive System:** *Cramp, flatulence, indigestion, nausea.*
**Nervous System:** *Depression, nervous exhaustion, neuralgia, tension, and stress.*

**EXTRACTION**
Essential oil by steam distillation from the leaves or the fruit. An oleoresin from the berries is also produced.

**ACTIONS**
Anesthetic, analgesic, antioxidant, antiseptic, carminative, muscle relaxant, rubefacient, stimulant, tonic.

**COMPATIBILITIES**
It blends well with ginger, geranium, lavender, opopanax, labdanum, ylang ylang, patchouli, orange blossom, oriental and spicy bases.

**SAFETY DATA**
*Contains eugenol, which irritates the mucous membranes, and has been found to cause dermal irritation. Pimenta leaf and berry oil should therefore be used with care in low dilutions only*

---

*PIMENTA RACEMOSA*

# West Indian bay

FAMILY: MYRTACEAE

### Herbal/Folk Tradition

The West Indian bay tree is often grown together with the allspice or pimento bush, then the fruits of both are dried and powdered to make household allspice. The bay leaves are distilled in rum to make the famous old hair tonic.

DRIED WEST
INDIAN BAY BARK

*A wild-growing tropical evergreen tree up to 26ft (8m) high, with large leathery leaves and aromatic fruits.*

## DATAFILE

**AROMATHERAPY/ HOME USE**

**Skin Care:** *Scalp stimulant, hair rinse for dandruff, greasy, lifeless hair, and promoting growth.*
**Circulation, Muscles, and Joints:** *Muscular and articular aches and pains, neuralgia, poor circulation, rheumatism, sprains, strains.*
**Immune System:** *Colds, flu, infectious diseases.*

**EXTRACTION**
Essential oil by water or steam distillation from the leaves. An oleoresin is also produced in small quantities.

**ACTIONS**
Analgesic, anticonvulsant, antineuralgic, expectorant, antirheumatic, antiseptic, astrigent, stimulant, tonic (for hair).

**COMPATIBILITIES**
It blends well with lavender, lavandin, rosemary, geranium, ylang ylang, citrus and spice oils.

**SAFETY DATA**
*Moderately toxic due to high eugenol content; a mucous membrane irritant, so use in moderation. Unlike bay laurel, however, it does not appear to cause dermal irritation or sensitization*

*PIMPINELLA ANISUM*

# Aniseed

FAMILY: APIACEAE (UMBELLIFERAE)

## Herbal/Folk Tradition

Widely used as a domestic spice. The volatile oil content provides the basis for its medicinal applications: dry irritable coughs, bronchitis, and whooping cough. Aniseed tea is used for infant catarrh, also flatulence, colic, and griping pains, painful periods and to promote breast milk.

ANISEED SEEDS

*An annual herb, less than 3ft (1m) high, with delicate leaves and white flowers.*

### DATAFILE

**AROMATHERAPY/ HOME USE**
See Star anise, page 90.

**EXTRACTION**
Essential oil by steam distillation from the seeds.

**ACTIONS**
Antiseptic, antispasmodic, carminative, diuretic, expectorant, galactagogue, stimulant, stomachic.

*Pimpinella anisum
Native to Greece and Egypt, now widely cultivated. In Turkey, a popular alcholoic drink, raki, is made from the seed.*

### SAFETY DATA
*Contains anethole, which is known to cause dermatitis – avoid in allergic and inflammatory skin conditions. In large doses it is narcotic and slows down the circulation; can lead to cerebral disorders. Use in moderation. Avoid during pregnancy*

---

*PINUS MUGO VAR. PUMILIO*

# Dwarf pine

FAMILY: PINACEAE

## Herbal/Folk Tradition

A preparation made from the needles has been used internally for bladder, kidney, and rheumatic complaints, as a liniment for rheumatism and muscular pain, and as an inhalant for bronchitis, catarrh, colds, etc.

DWARF PINE NEEDLES

*A pyramidal shrub or small tree up to 39ft (12m) high with a black bark, stiff and twisted needles borne in clusters, and brown cones, initially of a bluish hue.*

### DATAFILE

**AROMATHERAPY/ HOME USE**
None. It is best avoided therapeutically due to irritant hazards.

**EXTRACTION**
Essential oil by steam distillation from the needles and twigs.

**ACTIONS**
Analgesic, antimicrobial, antiseptic, antitussive, antiviral, balsamic, diuretic, expectorant, rubefacient.

**COMPATIBILITIES**
Its unique delicate odor blends well with cedarwood, lavandin,

*Pinus mugo var. pumilio
Native to the mountainous regions of central and southern Europe.*

rosemary, sage, cananga, labdanum, juniper, and other coniferous oils.

### SAFETY DATA
*Dermal irritant, common sensitizing agent; otherwise nontoxic*

*PINUS PALUSTRIS*

# Longleaf pine

FAMILY: PINACEAE

## Herbal/Folk Tradition

Pine sawdust has been used for centuries as a highly esteemed household remedy for a variety of ailments. It was valued as a powerful external antiseptic remedy, applied as a poultice.

FRESH PINE NEEDLES

STEM WITH BARK

*A tall evergreen tree with long needles and a straight trunk, grown for lumber. It exudes an oleoresin from the trunk, and is the largest turpentine source in the United States.*

### DATAFILE

**AROMATHERAPY/ HOME USE**

Circulation, Muscles, and Joints: *Arthritis, debility, lumbago, muscular aches and pains, poor circulation, rheumatism, stiffness, etc.*
Respiratory System: *Asthma, bronchitis, catarrh, sinusitis.*

**EXTRACTION**

The crude oil is obtained by steam distillation from the sawdust and wood chips from the heartwood and roots of the tree, and then submitted to fractional distillation under atmospheric pressure to produce pine essential oil.

**ACTIONS**

Analgesic (mild), antirheumatic, antiseptic, bactericidal, expectorant, insecticidal, stimulant.

**COMPATIBILITIES**

It blends well with rosemary, pine needle, cedarwood, citronella, rosewood, ho leaf, and oakmoss.

**SAFETY DATA**

*Nontoxic, nonirritant (except in concentration), possible sensitization in some individuals*

---

*PINUS PALUSTRIS AND OTHER PINUS SPECIES*

# Turpentine

FAMILY: PINACEAE

## Herbal/Folk Tradition

Known since ancient times for its application to genitourinary and pulmonary infections, digestive complaints, and externally for rheumatic or neuralgic pain and skin conditions.

FRESH TURPENTINE

*"Gum turpentine" is a term applied to the oleoresin formed as a physiological product in the trunks of various Pinus, Picea, and Abies species. Turpentine refers both to the crude oleoresin and to the distilled and rectified essential oils.*

### DATAFILE

**AROMATHERAPY/ HOME USE**

See Mastic, page 118.

**EXTRACTION**

Essential oil by steam (or water) distillation from the crude oleoresin, then rectified.

**ACTIONS**

Analgesic, antimicrobial, antirheumatic, antiseptic, antispasmodic, balsamic, diuretic, cicatrizant, counterirritant, expectorant, hemostatic, parasiticide, rubefacient, stimulant, tonic, vermifuge.

*Pinus elliottii*
*Produced all over the world, and widely used in ointments for aches and pains and in cough and cold remedies.*

**SAFETY DATA**

*Enviromental hazard – marine pollutant. Relatively nontoxic and nonirritant; possible sensitization in some individuals. Avoid therapeutic use or employ in moderation only*

*PINUS SYLVESTRIS*

# Scotch pine

FAMILY: PINACEAE

### Herbal/Folk Tradition

It was used by the Native Americans to prevent scurvy, and to stuff mattresses to repel lice and fleas. As an inhalation it helps relieve bronchial catarrh, asthma, blocked sinuses. The pine kernels are an excellent restorative.

FRESH NEEDLES

SCOTCH PINE CONE

*A tall evergreen tree, up to 131ft (40m) high with a flat crown. It has a reddish-brown, deeply fissured bark, long stiff needles that grow in pairs, and pointed brown cones.*

## DATAFILE

### AROMATHERAPY/ HOME USE

**Skin Care:** *Cuts, lice, excessive perspiration, scabies, sores.*
**Circulation, Muscles, and Joints:** *Arthritis, gout, muscular aches and pains, poor circulation, rheumatism.*
**Respiratory System:** *Asthma, bronchitis, catarrh, coughs, sinusitis.*
**Genitourinary System:** *Cystitis, urinary infection.*
**Immune System:** *Colds, flu.*
**Nervous System:** *Fatigue, nervous exhaustion, neuralgia.*

### EXTRACTION

Essential oil by dry distillation of the needles.

### ACTIONS

Antimicrobial, antineuralgic, antirheumatic, antiscorbutic, antiseptic (pulmonary, urinary, hepatic), antiviral, bactericidal, balsamic, cholagogue, choleretic, deodorant, diuretic, expectorant, hypertensive, insecticidal, restorative, rubefacient, stimulant (adrenal cortex, circulatory, nervous), vermifuge.

### COMPATIBILITIES

It blends well with cedarwood, rosemary, tea tree, sage, lavender, juniper, lemon, niaouli, eucalyptus, and marjoram.

### SAFETY DATA

Nontoxic, nonirritant (except in concentration), possible sensitization. Avoid in allergic skin conditions

---

*PIPER CUBEBA*

# Cubeb

FAMILY: PIPERACEAE

### Herbal/Folk Tradition

It has been traditionally used for treating genito-urinary infections, such as gonorrhea, cystitis, urethritis, abscess of the prostate gland, and leucorrhea. It is also used for digestive upsets and respiratory problems.

DRIED CUBEB SEED

*An evergreen climbing vine up to 20ft (6m) high with heart-shaped leaves. Altogether similar to the black pepper plant, except that the fruit or seeds of the cubeb retain their peduncle or stem – thus the name, tailed pepper.*

## DATAFILE

### AROMATHERAPY/ HOME USE

**Respiratory System:** *Bronchitis, catarrh, congestion, chronic coughs, sinusitis, throat infections.*
**Digestive System:** *Flatulence, indigestion, piles, sluggish digestion.*
**Genitourinary System:** *Cystitis, leucorrhea, urethritis.*

### EXTRACTION

Essential oil by steam distillation from the unripe but fully grown fruits or berries. An oleoresin is also produced in small quantities.

### ACTIONS

Antiseptic (pulmonary, genito-urinary), antispasmodic, antiviral, bactericidal, carminative, diuretic, expectorant, stimulant.

### COMPATIBILITIES

It blends well with cananga, galbanum, lavender, rosemary, black pepper, allspice, and other spices.

### SAFETY DATA

Nontoxic, nonirritant, nonsensitizing. Frequently subject to adulteration

*PIPER NIGRUM*

# Black pepper

FAMILY: PIPERACEAE

## Herbal/Folk Tradition

Both black and white pepper have been used
in the East for over 4,000 years for medicinal
and culinary purposes.
In China, white
pepper is used to
treat malaria,
cholera, dysentery,
diarrhea, stomach-
ache, and other
digestive problems.

DRIED PEPPERCORN

FRUIT

FRESH CUTTING

*A perennial woody vine up to 16ft (5m) high with heart-
shaped leaves and white flowers. Berries mature from red to
black – black pepper is the fully grown, unripe fruit.*

### DATAFILE

**AROMATHERAPY/
HOME USE**
Not compatible with
homeopathic treatment.
**Skin Care:** *Chilblains.*
**Circulation, Muscles, and Joints:**
*Anemia, arthritis, muscular aches
and pains, neuralgia, poor
circulation, poor muscle tone
(muscular atonia), rheumatic pain,
sprains, stiffness.*
**Respiratory System:** *Catarrh,
chills.*
**Digestive System:** *Colic,
constipation, diarrhea, flatulence,
heartburn, loss of appetite, nausea.*
**Immune System:** *Colds, flu,
infections, and viruses.*

**EXTRACTION**
Essential oil by steam distillation
from dried black peppercorns.

**ACTIONS**
Analgesic, antimicrobial,
antiseptic, antispasmodic,
antitoxic, aperitif, aphrodisiac,
bactericidal, carminative,
diaphoretic, digestive, diuretic,
febrifuge, laxative, rubefacient,
stimulant (nervous, circulatory,
digestive), stomachic, tonic.

**COMPATIBILITIES**
Frankincense, sandalwood,
lavender, rosemary, marjoram,
spices, and florals.

**SAFETY DATA**
*Nontoxic, nonsensitizing, irritant in high concentration due
to rubefacient properties. Use in moderation only*

---

*PISTACIA LENTISCUS*

# Mastic

FAMILY: ANACARDIACEAE

## Herbal/Folk Tradition

In the East it is used in the manufacture
of confectionery and
cordials; it is still
used medicinally
for diarrhea in
children and to
sweeten the
breath. The oil
was used in the
West in a similar
way to turpentine.

FRESH MASTIC

*A small bushy tree or shrub up to 10ft (3m) high, which
produces a natural oleoresin from the trunk. Incisions are
made in the bark in order to collect the liquid oleoresin,
which then hardens into brittle pea-size lumps.*

### DATAFILE

**AROMATHERAPY/
HOME USE**
Use with care for:
**Skin Care:** *Boils, cuts, fleas, insect
repellant, lice, ringworm, scabies,
wounds.*
**Circulation, Muscles, and Joints:**
*Arthritis, gout, muscular aches and
pains, rheumatism, sciatica.*
**Respiratory System:** *Bronchitis,
catarrh, whooping cough.*
**Genitourinary System:**
*Cystitis, leucorrhea, urethritis.*
**Immune System:** *Colds.*
**Nervous System:** *Neuralgia.*

**EXTRACTION**
A resinoid is produced by
solvent extraction from the
oleoresin, and an essential oil is
produced by steam distillation
from the oleoresin.

**ACTIONS**
Antimicrobial, antiseptic,
antispasmodic, astringent,
diuretic, expectorant, stimulant.

**COMPATIBILITIES**
Lavender, mimosa, and citrus
and floral oils.

**SAFETY DATA**
*Nontoxic, nonirritant, possible sensitization in some individuals*

*POGOSTEMON CABLIN*

# Patchouli

FAMILY: LAMIACEAE (LABIATAE)

## Herbal/Folk Tradition

The oil is used in the East to scent
linen and clothes,
and it is believed
to help prevent
the spread of
disease. In China,
Japan, and
Malaysia the herb
is used to treat
colds, headaches,
nausea, diarrhea,
abdominal pain,
and halitosis.

FRESH PATCHOULI

*A perennial bushy herb up to 3ft (1m) high with a sturdy,
hairy stem, large, fragrant, furry leaves, and white flowers
tinged with purple.*

### DATAFILE

**AROMATHERAPY/
HOME USE**
Skin Care: *Acne, athlete's foot,
cracked and chapped skin,
dandruff, dermatitis, eczema
(weeping), fungal infections,
impetigo, insect repellent, oily hair
and skin, open pores, sores,
wounds, wrinkles.*
Nervous System: *Frigidity, nervous
exhaustion, and stress.*

**EXTRACTION**
Essential oil by steam distillation
of the dried leaves.

**ACTIONS**
Antidepressant, anti-inflammatory,
antiemetic, antimicrobial,
antiphlogistic, antiseptic, antitoxic,
antiviral, aphrodisiac, astringent,
bactericidal, carminative,
cicatrizant, deodorant, digestive,
diuretic, febrifuge, fungicidal,
nervine, prophylactic, stimulant
(nervous), stomachic, tonic.

**COMPATIBILITIES**
Labdanum, vetiver, sandalwood,
cedarwood, oakmoss, geranium,
clove, lavender, rose, orange
blossom, cassia, bergamot,
myrrh, clary sage, opopanax,
and oriental bases.

**SAFETY DATA**
*Nontoxic, nonirritant, nonsensitizing*

---

*POLIANTHES TUBEROSA*

# Tuberose

FAMILY: AGAVACEAE

## Herbal/Folk Tradition

The double-flowered variety is grown
for ornamental
purposes and for use
by the cut flower
trade. The pure
absolute extraction of
tuberose is one of the
most expensive
natural flower oils at
the disposal of the
modern perfumer.

FRESH
TUBEROSE LEAVES

*A tender, tall, slim perennial up to 20in (50cm) high, with
long slender leaves, a tuberous root, and large, very
fragrant, white lilylike flowers.*

### DATAFILE

**AROMATHERAPY/
HOME USE**
Used in high-quality perfumes,

**EXTRACTION**
A concrete and absolute by
solvent extraction from the
fresh flowers, picked before the
petals open. (An essential oil is
also obtained by distillation of
the concrete.)

**ACTIONS**
Narcotic.

**COMPATIBILITIES**
Gardenia, violet, opopanax, rose,
jasmine, carnation, orris, Peru
balsam, orange blossom, and
ylang ylang.

*Polianthes tuberosa*

**SAFETY DATA**
*No safety data available – often adulterated*

*PRUNUS DULCIS VAR. AMARA*

# Bitter almond

FAMILY: ROSACEAE

### Herbal/Folk Tradition

A "fixed" oil commonly known as "sweet almond oil" is made by pressing the kernels from both the sweet and bitter almond trees. It is used as a laxative, for bronchitis, heartburn, coughs, and disorders of the kidneys, bladder, and biliary ducts.

BITTER ALMOND KERNELS

*The almond tree grows to a height of about 7m (23ft) and has pinky-white blossom. It is classified as a drupe.*

### DATAFILE

**AROMATHERAPY/ HOME USE**
None. It should not be used therapeutically, either internally or externally.

**EXTRACTION**
Essential oil by steam distillation from the kernels. The nuts are pressed and macerated in warm water for 12–24 hours before the oil is extracted. It is during this process that the prussic acid is formed; it is not present in the raw seed. Most commercial bitter almond oil is rectified to remove all prussic acid.

*Bitter almond*

**ACTIONS**
Anesthetic, antispasmodic, narcotic, vermifuge (FFPA).

**SAFETY DATA**
*Prussic acid, also known as hydrocyanic acid or cyanide, is a well-known poison. Benzaldehyde is also moderately toxic*

---

*ROSA X CENTIFOLIA*

# Cabbage rose

FAMILY: ROSACEAE

### Herbal/Folk Tradition

Up to the Middle Ages the rose was an essential remedy, used for a wide range of disorders, from digestive and menstrual problems to headaches, fever (plague), eye infections, and skin complaints.

DRIED ROSE BUDS

*The rose that is generally used for oil production is strictly a hybrid involving R. x centifolia, R. gallica, and a few other roses. Known as* rose de mai, *it grows to 8ft (2.5m) high and has a mass of pink or rosy-purple flowers.*

### DATAFILE

**AROMATHERAPY/ HOME USE**
See Damask rose, page 121.

**EXTRACTION**
See Damask rose, page 121.

**ACTIONS**
See Damask rose, page 121.

**COMPATIBILITIES**
It blends well with jasmine, cassie, mimosa, orange blossom, geranium, bergamot, lavender, clary sage, sandalwood, guaiacwood, patchouli, benzoin, chamomile, Peru balsam, clove, and palmarosa.

**SAFETY DATA**
*Nontoxic, nonirritant, nonsensitizing*

*ROSA X DAMASCENA*

# Damask rose

FAMILY: ROSACEAE

DAMASK ROSE PETALS

## Herbal/Folk Tradition

Culpepers's *Complete Herbal* indicates that "oil of roses is used by itself to cool hot inflammations or swellings, and to bind and stay fluxes of humours to sores."[23] Rose hips are still current in the British Herbal Pharmacopoeia, mainly because of their high vitamin C content. See also Cabbage rose, page 120.

*The essential oil is a pale yellow or olive yellow liquid with a very rich, deep, sweet-floral, slightly spicy scent.*

*Small prickly shrub between 3–6ft (1–2m) high, with pink fragrant blooms and whitish hairy leaves.*

---

**DATAFILE**

### AROMATHERAPY/ HOME USE

**Skin Care:** *Broken capillaries, conjunctivitis (rose water), dry skin, eczema, herpes, mature and sensitive complexions, wrinkles.*
**Circulation, Muscles, and Joints:** *Palpitations, poor circulation.*
**Respiratory System:** *Asthma, coughs, hay fever.*
**Digestive System:** *Cholecystitis, liver congestion, nausea.*
**Genitourinary System:** *Irregular menstruation, leucorrhea, menorrhagia, uterine disorders.*
**Nervous System:** *Depression, impotence, insomnia, frigidity, headache, nervous tension, and stress-related complaints. The*

*rose, traditionally associated with Venus, the goddess of love and beauty, induces a feeling of well-being and happiness.*

### EXTRACTION

Essential oil by water or steam distillation from the fresh petals. Rose water is produced as a by-product of this process. Concrete and absolute by solvent extraction from the fresh petals. A rose leaf absolute is also produced in small quantities in France.

*Damask rose*

### ACTIONS

Antidepressant, antiphlogistic, antiseptic, antispasmodic, anti-tubercular agent, antiviral, aphrodisiac, astringent, bactericidal, choleretic, cicatrizant, depurative, emmenagogue, hemostatic, hepatic, laxative, regulator of appetite, sedative (nervous), stomachic, tonic (heart, liver, stomach, uterus).

### COMPATIBILITIES

It blends well with most oils and is useful for "rounding off" blends. The Bulgarian type is considered superior in perfumery work.

---

**SAFETY DATA**
*Nontoxic, nonirritant, nonsensitizing*

*ROSMARINUS OFFICINALIS*

# Rosemary

FAMILY: LAMIACEAE (LABIATAE)

FRESH ROSEMARY

## Herbal/Folk Tradition

One of the earliest plants to be used for food, medicine, and magic. Sprigs of rosemary were burned at shrines in ancient Greece, fumigations were used in the Middle Ages to drive away evil spirits and as a protection against plague.

It has been used for a wide range of complaints including respiratory and circulatory disorders, liver congestion, digestive and nervous complaints, muscular and rheumatic pain, skin and hair problems. It is current in the *British Herbal Pharmacopoeia* as a specific for "depressive states with general debility and indications of cardiovascular weakness".[24]

*A shrubby evergreen bush up to 6ft (2m) high, with silvery-green, needle-shaped leaves and pale blue flowers. The whole plant is strongly aromatic.*

**DATAFILE**

### AROMATHERAPY HOME USE

**Skin Care:** *Acne, dandruff, dermatitis, eczema, greasy hair, insect repellent, lice, promotes hair growth, regulates seborrhea, scabies, stimulates scalp, varicose veins.*

**Circulation, Muscles, and Joints:** *Arteriosclerosis, fluid retention, gout, muscular pain, palpitations, poor circulation, rheumatism.*

**Respiratory System:** *Asthma, bronchitis, whooping cough.*

**Digestive System:** *Colitis, dyspepsia, flatulence, hepatic disorders, hypercholesterolemia, jaundice.*

**Genitourinary System:** *Dysmenorrhea, leucorrhea.*

**Immune System:** *Colds, flu, infections.*

**Nervous System:** *Debility, headaches, hypotension, neuralgia, mental fatigue, nervous exhaustion, and stress-related disorders.*

### EXTRACTION

Essential oil by steam distillation of the fresh flowering tops or (in Spain) the whole plant (poorer quality).

### ACTIONS

Analgesic, antimicrobial, antioxidant, antirheumatic, antiseptic, antispasmodic, aphrodisiac, astringent, carminative, cephalic, cholagogue, choleretic, cicatrizant, cordial, cytophylactic, diaphoretic, digestive, diuretic, emmenagogue, fungicidal, hepatic, hypertensive, nervine, parasiticide, restorative, rubefacient, stimulant (circulatory, adrenal cortex, hepatobiliary), stomachic, sudorific, tonic (nervous, general), vulnerary.

### COMPATIBILITIES

It blends well with olibanum, lavender, lavandin, citronella, oregano, thyme, pine, basil, peppermint, labdanum, elemi, cedarwood, petitgrain, cinnamon, and other spice oils.

**SAFETY DATA**

*Nontoxic, nonirritant (in dilution only), nonsensitizing. Avoid during pregnancy. Not to be used by epileptics. Contraindicated in cases of high blood pressure*

*RUTA GRAVEOLENS*

# Rue

FAMILY: RUTACEAE

## Herbal/Folk Tradition

A favored remedy of the ancients, especially as an antidote to poison. It was seen as a magic herb by many cultures and as a protection against evil. It was also used for nervous afflictions.

FRESH RUE

*An ornamental, shrubby herb with a strong, aromatic, bitter, or acrid scent. It has tough, woody branches, small, smooth, bluish-green leaves, and greeny-yellow flowers.*

### DATAFILE

**AROMATHERAPY/ HOME USE**
None. It should not be used in aromatherapy.

**EXTRACTION**
Essential oil by steam distillation from the fresh herb.

**ACTIONS**
Antitoxic, antitussive, antiseptic, antispasmodic, diuretic, emmenagogue, insecticidal, nervine, rubefacient, stimulant, tonic, vermifuge.

*Ruta graveolens*
*Native to the Mediterranean, found growing wild in Spain, Morocco, Corsica, Sardinia, and Algeria.*

### SAFETY DATA
*Oral toxin (due to main constituent). Skin and mucous membrane irritant. Abortifacient. "Rue oil should never be used in perfumery or flavor work."[25]*

---

*SALVIA LAVANDULIFOLIA*

# Spanish sage

FAMILY: LAMIACEAE (LABIATAE)

## Herbal/Folk Tradition

In Spain it is regarded as a "cure-all". Believed to promote longevity and protect against infection. Used for rheumatism, digestive complaints, menstrual problems, infertility, and nervous weakness.

SMALL PURPLE FLOWERS

FRESH LEAF

*An evergreen shrub, similar to the garden sage but with narrower leaves and small purple flowers. The whole plant is aromatic with a scent reminiscent of spike lavender.*

### DATAFILE

**AROMATHERAPY/ HOME USE**
Skin Care: *Acne, cuts, dandruff, dermatitis, eczema, gingivitis gum infections, hair loss, sores, sweating.*
Circulation, Muscles, and Joints: *Arthritis, debility, fluid retention, muscular aches, poor circulation, rheumatism.*
Respiratory System: *Asthma, coughs, laryngitis.*
Digestive System: *Jaundice, liver congestion.*
Genitourinary System: *Amenorrhea, dysmenorrhea,*
Immune System: *Colds, flu.*
Nervous System: *Headaches, nervous exhaustion, and stress.*

**EXTRACTION**
Essential oil by steam distillation.

**ACTIONS**
Antidepressant, anti-inflammatory, antimicrobial, antiseptic, antispasmodic, astringent, carminative, deodorant, depurative, digestive, emmenagogue, expectorant, febrifuge, hypotensive, nervine, regulator (of seborrhea), stimulant (hepatobiliary, adrenocortical glands, circulation), stomachic, tonic (nerve and general).

**COMPATIBILITIES**
Rosemary, lavender, pine, clary sage, citronella, eucalyptus.

### SAFETY DATA
*Relatively nontoxic, nonirritant, nonsensitizing. Avoid during pregnancy; use in moderation*

# Common sage

FAMILY: LAMIACEAE (LABIATAE)

### Herbal/Folk Tradition

A herb of ancient repute, valued as a culinary and medicinal plant. It has been used for disorders including respiratory infections, menstrual difficulties, and digestive complaints. It was believed to strengthen the senses and memory.

FRESH COMMON SAGE

*An evergreen, shrubby, perennial herb up to 32in (80cm) high with a woody base, soft, silver, oval leaves, and a mass of deep blue or violet flowers.*

| DATAFILE | |
|---|---|
| **AROMATHERAPY/ HOME USE** <br> None. Use with care or avoid in therapeutic work altogether – Spanish sage or clary sage are good alternatives. <br><br> **EXTRACTION** <br> Essential oil by steam distillation from the dried leaves. A so-called oleoresin is also produced from the exhausted plant material. | **ACTIONS** <br> Anti-inflammatory, antimicrobial, antioxidant, antiseptic, antispasmodic, astringent, digestive, diuretic, emmenagogue, febrifuge, hypertensive, insecticidal, laxative, stomachic, tonic. <br><br> **COMPATIBILITIES** <br> It blends well with lavandin, rosemary, rosewood, lavender, hyssop, lemon, and other citrus oils. |

**SAFETY DATA**
*Oral toxin (due to thujone). Abortifacient; avoid in pregnancy. Avoid in epilepsy. Contraindicated in cases of high blood pressure*

# Clary sage

FAMILY: LAMIACEAE (LABIATAE)

### Herbal/Folk Tradition

This herb was highly esteemed in the Middle Ages and was used for digestive disorders, kidney disease, uterine and menstrual complaints, for cleansing ulcers, and as a general nerve tonic.

FRESH LEAF

*Stout biennial or perennial herb up to 3ft (1m) high with large, hairy leaves, green with a hint of purple, and small blue flowers.*

| DATAFILE | |
|---|---|
| **AROMATHERAPY/ HOME USE** <br> **Skin Care:** *Acne, boils, dandruff, hair loss, inflammation, oily skin, ophthalmia, ulcers, wrinkles.* <br> **Circulation, Muscles, and Joints:** *High blood pressure, muscular aches and pains.* <br> **Respiratory System:** *Asthma, throat infections.* <br> **Digestive System:** *Cramp, dyspepsia, flatulence.* <br> **Genitourinary System:** *Amenorrhea, labor pain, dysmenorrhea, leucorrhea.* <br> **Nervous System:** *Depression, frigidity, impotence, migraine, nervous tension, and stress.* | **EXTRACTION** <br> Essential oil by steam distillation from flowering tops and leaves. <br><br> **ACTIONS** <br> Anticonvulsive, antidepressant, antiphlogistic, antiseptic, anti-spasmodic, aphrodisiac, astringent, bactericidal, carminative, cicatrizant, deodorant, digestive, emmenagogue, euphoric, hypotensive, nervine, sedative, stomachic, tonic, uterine. <br><br> **COMPATIBILITIES** <br> Juniper, lavender, cilantro, pine, cardomon, geranium, sandalwood, jasmine, frankincense, and citrus oils. |

**SAFETY DATA**
*Nontoxic, nonirritant, nonsensitizing. Avoid during pregnancy. Do not use clary sage oil while drinking alcohol; it can induce a narcotic effect*

*SANTALUM ALBUM*

# Sandalwood

FAMILY: SANTALACEAE

### Herbal/Folk Tradition

One of the oldest known perfume materials, used for at least 4,000 years as a cosmetic and perfume all over the East. The Chinese use it to treat stomachache, gonorrhea, choleraic difficulties, and skin complaints.

SANDALWOOD CHIPPINGS

*A small evergreen, parasitic tree up to 30ft (9m) high with brown-gray trunk and many smooth, slender branches. It has leathery leaves and small pinky-purple flowers.*

### DATAFILE

#### AROMATHERAPY/HOME USE

**Skin Care:** *Acne, dry, cracked, and chapped skin, aftershave (barber's rash), greasy skin, moisturizer.*
**Respiratory System:** *Bronchitis, catarrh, dry coughs, laryngitis, sore throat.*
**Digestive System:** *Diarrhea, nausea.*
**Genitourinary System:** *Cystitis.*
**Nervous System:** *Depression, insomnia, nervous tension, and stress-related complaints.*

#### EXTRACTION

Essential oil by water or steam distillation from the roots and heartwood, powdered and dried.

#### ACTIONS

Antidepressant, antiphlogistic, antiseptic (urinary/pulmonary), antispasmodic, aphrodisiac, astringent, bactericidal, carminative, cicatrizant, diuretic, expectorant, insecticidal, sedative, tonic.

#### COMPATIBILITIES

Rose, violet, tuberose, clove, lavender, black pepper, bergamot, rosewood, mimosa, geranium, labdanum, oakmoss, benzoin, vetiver, patchouli, cassie, costus, myrrh, jasmine.

#### SAFETY DATA

Nontoxic, nonirritant, nonsensitizing

---

*SANTOLINA CHAMAECYPARISSUS*

# Santolina

FAMILY: ASTERACEAE (COMPOSITAE)

### Herbal/Folk Tradition

It was used as an antidote to all sorts of poison, and to expel worms. It was used to keep away moths from linen, to repel mosquitoes, and as a remedy for insect bits, warts, scabs, and plantar warts (verruccae).

FRESH SANTOLINA LEAVES

*An evergreen, woody shrub with whitish-gray foliage and small, bright yellow, ball-shaped flowers borne on long single stalks. The whole plant has a strong rank odor, a bit like chamomile.*

### DATAFILE

#### AROMATHERAPY/HOME USE

None. No safety data is currently available. It is likely to be highly toxic.

#### EXTRACTION

Essential oil by steam distillation from the seeds.

#### ACTIONS

Antispasmodic, antitoxic, anthelmintic, insecticidal, stimulant, vermifuge.

*Santolina chamaecyparissus Native to Italy, now common throughout the Mediterranean region. Much grown as a popular border herb.*

#### SAFETY DATA

Oral toxin

*SASSAFRAS ALBIDUM*

# Sassafras

FAMILY: LAURACEAE

## Herbal/Folk Tradition

It has been used for treating high blood pressure, rheumatism, arthritis, gout, menstrual and kidney problems, and for skin complaints. The wood and bark yield a bright yellow dye.

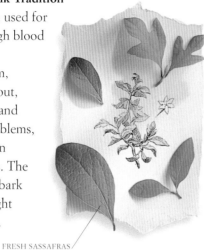

FRESH SASSAFRAS

*A deciduous tree up to 131ft (40m) high with many slender branches, a soft and spongy orange-brown bark, and small yellowy-green flowers. The bark and wood are aromatic.*

### DATAFILE

**AROMATHERAPY/ HOME USES**
None. It should not be used in therapy, either internally or externally.

**EXTRACTION**
Essential oil by steam distillation from the dried root bark chips.

**ACTIONS**
Antiviral, diaphoretic, diuretic, carminative, pediculicide (destroys lice), stimulant.

*Sassafras albidum*
*Native to eastern parts of the United States; the oil is produced mainly from Florida to Canada and in Mexico.*

**SAFETY DATA**
*Highly toxic – ingestion of even small amounts has been known to cause death. Carcinogen. Irritant. Abortifacient*

*SATUREJA HORTENSIS*

# Summer savory

FAMILY: LAMIACEAE (LABIATAE)

## Herbal/Folk Tradition

A popular culinary herb, with a peppery flavor. It has been used as a tea for various ailments including digestive and respiratory complaints and menstrual disorders. Used externally, the leaves bring relief from insect bites.

FRESH LEAF OF SUMMER SAVORY

*An annual herb up to 18in (45cm) high with slender, erect, slightly hairy stems, linear leaves and small, pale lilac flowers.*

### DATAFILE

**AROMATHERAPY/ HOME USE**
None. It should not be used on the skin.

**EXTRACTION**
Essential oil by steam distillation from the whole dried herb. An oleoresin is also produced by solvent extraction.

**ACTIONS**
Anticatarrhal, antiputrescent, antispasmodic, aphrodisiac, astringent, bactericidal, carminative, cicatrizant, emmenagogue, expectorant, fungicidal, stimulant, vermifuge.

**COMPATIBILITIES**
It blends well with lavender, lavandin, pine needle, oakmoss, rosemary, and citrus oils.

**SAFETY DATA**
*Dermal toxin, dermal irritant, mucous membrane irritant. Avoid during pregnancy*

*SATUREJA MONTANA*

# Winter savory

FAMILY: LAMIACEAE (LABIATAE)

## Herbal/Folk Tradition

It has been used as a culinary herb since
antiquity, much in the same way as
summer savory. It
was used as a
digestive remedy,
especially good
for colic, and in
Germany it is
used particularly
for diarrhea.

FRESH SPRIG OF
WINTER SAVORY

*A bushy perennial subshrub up to 16in (40cm) high
with woody stems at the base, linear leaves, and pale
purple flowers.*

### DATAFILE

**AROMATHERAPY/
HOME USE**
None. It should not be used on
the skin.

**EXTRACTION**
Essential oil by steam distillation
from the whole herb. Oleoresin
is produced by solvent
extraction.

**ACTIONS**
Anticatarrhal, antiputrescent,
antispasmodic, aphrodisiac,
astringent, bactericidal,
carminative, cicatrizant,
emmenagogue, expectorant,
fungicidal, stimulant, vermifuge.

*Satureja montana
Native to the Mediterranean
region, now found all over
Europe, Russia and Turkey.*

**SAFETY DATA**
See Summer savory, page 126

---

*SAUSSUREA COSTUS*

# Costus

FAMILY: ASTERACEA (COMPOSITAE)

## Herbal/Folk Tradition

The root has been used for millennia
in India and China
for digestive
complaints,
respiratory
conditions, as a
stimulant, and
for infection
including typhoid
and cholera. It
is also used as an
incense.

DRIED LEAVES

*A large, erect, perennial plant up to 6ft (2m) high with a
thick, tapering root and numerous almost black flowers.*

### DATAFILE

**AROMATHERAPY/
HOME USE**
Costus is not recommended for
aromatherapy or home use
because it is a common and
severe dermal sensitizer. In a
recent skin test, it produced
sensitization reactions in all 25
volunteers.

**EXTRACTION**
The dried roots are macerated
in warm water, then subjected
to steam distillation followed by
solvent extraction of the
distilled water. (A concrete and
absolute are also produced in
small quantities.)

**ACTIONS**
Antiseptic, antispasmodic,
antiviral, bactericidal,
carminative, digestive,
expectorant, febrifuge,
hypotensive, stimulant,
stomachic, tonic.

**COMPATIBILITIES**
Patchouli, ylang ylang, opopanax,
and oriental and floral
fragrances.

**SAFETY DATA**
Although costus is classified as nontoxic and nonirritant,
it is a severe dermal sensitizer

ESSENTIAL OILS

## SCHINUS MOLLE

# Schinus molle

FAMILY: ANACARDIACEAE

### Herbal/Folk Tradition

In Greece and other Mediterranean countries an intoxicating beverage is made from the fruits of the tree. The fruit is used as a substitute for black pepper; this happened during World War II, when black pepper oil was unavailable.

FRESH LEAVES

*A tropical evergreen tree up to 65ft (20m) high, with graceful, drooping branches, feathery foliage and fragrant yellow flowers. The berries or fruit have an aromatic, peppery flavor.*

### DATAFILE

**AROMATHERAPY/ HOME USE**
Not compatible with homeopathic treatment.
**Skin Care:** *Chilblains.*
**Circulation, Muscles, and Joints:** *Anemia, arthritis, muscular ache, neuralgia, poor circulation, poor muscle tone, rheumatic pain, stiffness.*
**Respiratory System:** *Catarrh, chills.*
**Digestive System:** *Appetite loss, colic, constipation, nausea, diarrhea, flatulence, heartburn,*
**Immune System:** *Colds, flu, infections, and viruses.*

**EXTRACTION**
Essential oil by steam distillation from the fruit or berries. An oil from the leaf is produced in small quantities.

**ACTIONS**
Antiseptic, antiviral, bactericidal, carminative, stimulant, stomachic.

**COMPATIBILITIES**
It blends well with oakmoss, clove, nutmeg, cinnamon, black pepper, and eucalyptus.

**SAFETY DATA**
*Nontoxic, nonirritant, nonsensitizing*

## SPARTIUM JUNCEUM

# Spanish broom

FAMILY: FABACEAE (LEGUMINOSAE)

### Herbal/Folk Tradition

Spanish broom has similar, but stronger, therapeutic properties to those of common broom, used to treat cardiac dropsy, myocardial weakness, tachycardia, and profuse menstruation.

PEA-LIKE FRAGRANT FLOWERS

*A decorative plant, up to 10ft (3m) high with upright woody branches and tough flexible stems. It has bright green leaves and large, yellow, pealike fragrant flowers, also bearing its seed pods or legumes.*

### DATAFILE

**AROMATHERAPY/ HOME USE**
None. In large doses, it causes vomiting, renal irritation, weakens the heart, depresses the nerve cells, and lowers the blood pressure, and in extreme cases causes death.

**EXTRACTION**
An absolute is obtained by solvent extraction from the dried flowers.

**ACTIONS**
Antihemorrhagic, cardioactive, diuretic, cathartic, emmenagogue, narcotic, vasoconstrictor.

*Spartium junceum*

**COMPATIBILITIES**
It blends well with rose, tuberose, cassie, mimosa, violet, vetiver, and herbaceous-type fragrances.

**SAFETY DATA**
*Sparteine, contained in the flowers as the main active constituent, is toxic*

*STYRAX BENZOIN*

# Benzoin

FAMILY: STYRACACEAE

## Herbal/Folk Tradition

Used for thousands of years in the East as a medicine and incense. In the West, best known as the compound tincture friars balsam, used for respiratory complaints. Externally it is used for cuts and irritable skin; used internally to aid digestion.

BENZOIN RESIN

*A large tropical tree up to 65ft (20m) high with pale green citruslike leaves, whitish underneath, bearing hard-shelled flattish fruit.*

### DATAFILE

**AROMATHERAPY/HOME USE**

**Skin Care:** *Cuts, chapped skin, inflammations, and irritations.*
**Circulation, Muscles, and Joints:** *Arthritis, gout, poor circulation, rheumatism.*
**Respiratory System:** *Asthma, bronchitis, colic, coughs, laryngitis.*
**Immune System:** *Flu.*
**Nervous System:** *Nervous tension.*

**EXTRACTION**

Crude benzoin is collected directly from the trees. Benzoin resinoid is prepared from the crude using solvents.

**ACTIONS**

Anti-inflammatory, antioxidant, antiseptic, astringent, carminative, cordial, deodorant, diuretic, expectorant, sedative, styptic, vulnerary.

**COMPATIBILITIES**

Blends well with sandalwood, rose, jasmine, myrrh, cypress, juniper, lemon, cilantro, and other spice oils.

### SAFETY DATA

*Nontoxic, nonirritant, possible sensitization. Compound benzoin tincture is "regarded as moderately toxic, due probably to occasional contact dermatitis developed in some individuals ... which contains, in addition to benzoin, aloe, storax, Tolu balsam and others."[26]*

---

*SYZYGIUM AROMATICUM*

# Clove

FAMILY: MYRTACEAE

## Herbal/Folk Tradition

Used as a domestic spice worldwide. Tincture of cloves has been used for skin infections, digestive upsets, for intestinal parasites; to ease the pain of childbirth, and toothache.

DRIED CLOVES

*A slender evergreen tree up to 39ft (12m) high. Its bright green leaves stand in pairs on short stalks. The long buds have a rosy-pink corolla at the tip; as the corolla fades the calyx turns red. These are beaten from the tree and dried.*

### DATAFILE

**AROMATHERAPY/HOME USE**

Only use clove bud oil.
**Skin Care:** *Acne, athlete's foot, bruises, burns, cuts, mosquito repellent, toothache, ulcers.*
**Circulation, Muscles, and Joints:** *Arthritis, rheumatism, sprains.*
**Respiratory System:** *Asthma, bronchitis.*
**Digestive System:** *Colic, nausea.*
**Immune System:** *Colds, flu,*

**EXTRACTION**

Essential oil by water distillation from buds or eaves, or by steam distillation from stalks or stems.

**ACTIONS**

Anthelmintic, antibiotic, anti-aphrodisiac, emetic, antihistaminic, antirheumatic, antineuralgic, antioxidant, antiseptic, antiviral, , carminative, counter-irritant, expectorant, larvicidal, stimulant, spasmolytic, stomachic, vermifuge.

**COMPATIBILITIES**

Rose, lavender, vanillin, clary sage, bergamot, bay leaf, lavandin, allspice, ylang ylang, and cananga.

### SAFETY DATA

*All clove oil can cause skin and mucous membrane irritation; clove bud and stem oil may cause dermatitis. Clove bud is the least toxic of the tree oils because of the lower eugenol percentage. Use in moderation only, in low dilution (less than 1 per cent)*

TAGETES MINUTA

# Tagetes

FAMILY: ASTERACEAE (COMPOSITAE)

### Herbal/Folk Tradition

In China the flowers of the African marigold are used for whooping cough, colds, colic, mumps, sore eyes, and mastitis. In India flowering tops of French marigold are distilled into a solvent, such as sandalwood oil, to make a perfume.

FRESH TAGETES FLOWER

*A strongly scented annual herb about 12in (30cm) high with bright orange, daisylike flowers and green oval leaves.*

DATAFILE

**AROMATHERAPY/ HOME USE**
Skin Care: *Bunions, calluses, corns, fungal infections.*

**EXTRACTION**
An essential oil by steam distillation from the fresh flowering herb. An absolute and concrete by solvent extraction from the fresh flowering herb.

**ACTIONS**
Anthelmintic, antispasmodic, bactericidal, carminative, diaphoretic, emmenagogue, fungicidal, stomachic.

*Tagetes minuta*
*Native to South America and Mexico.*

**COMPATIBILITIES**
It blends well with clary sage, lavender, jasmine, bergamot, and other citrus oils in very small percentages.

**SAFETY DATA**
*"It is quite possible that 'tagetone' (the main constituent) is harmful to the human organism."[27] Some reported cases of dermatitis with the tagetes species. Use with care, in moderation*

---

TANACETUM VULGARE

# Tansy

FAMILY: ASTERACEAE (COMPOSITAE)

### Herbal/Folk Tradition

FRESH TANSY

It has a long history of medicinal use, especially among gypsies, and is regarded as a "cure-all". It was used to expel worms, to treat colds and fever, prevent miscarriage, and ease dyspepsia.

*A hardy perennial wayside herb, up to 3ft (1m) high, with a smooth stem, dark ferny leaves, and small, round brilliant yellow flowers borne in clusters. The whole plant is strongly scented.*

DATAFILE

**AROMATHERAPY/ HOME USE**
None. It should not be used in aromatherapy, either internally or externally.

**EXTRACTION**
Essential oil by steam distillation from the whole herb (aerial parts).

**ACTIONS**
Anthelmintic, anti-inflammatory, antispasmodic, carminative, diaphoretic, digestive, emmenagogue, febrifuge, nervine, stimulant, tonic, vermifuge.

*Tanacetum vulgare*
*Native to central Europe, nationalized in North America, and now found in most temperate regions of the world.*

**SAFETY DATA**
*Oral toxin – due to high thujone content. Abortifacient*

*THUJA OCCIDENTALIS*

# Thuja

FAMILY: CUPRESSACEAE

### Herbal/Folk Tradition

Used as an incense by ancient civilizations. A decoction of leaves has been used for coughs, fever, intestinal parasites, venereal diseases, and cystitis. The ointment has been used for rheumatism, gout, warts, and plantar warts (verrucae).

THUJA SEEDS

*A pyramid-shaped coniferous tree up to 65ft (20m) high with scalelike leaves and broadly winged seeds. The tree must be fifteen years old before it is used for oil production.*

### DATAFILE

**AROMATHERAPY/ HOME USE**
None. It should not be used in aromatherapy, either internally or externally.

**EXTRACTION**
Essential oil by steam distillation from the leaves, twigs, and bark.

**ACTIONS**
Antirheumatic, astringent, diuretic, emmenagogue, expectorant, insect repellent, rubefacient, stimulant (nerves, uterus, and heart muscles), tonic, vermifuge.

*Thuja occidentalis*
*Native to northeastern North America; cultivated in France. The oil is produced mainly in Canada and the United States.*

**SAFETY DATA**
Oral toxin – poisonous due to high thujone content. Abortifacient

---

*THYMUS CAPITATUS*

# Spanish oregano

FAMILY: LAMIACEAE (LABIATAE)

### Herbal/Folk Tradition

The properties and oil of Spanish oregano (*Thymus capitatus*) are similar to the common thyme (*T. vulgaris*); it also shares many qualities with common oregano or wild marjoram (*Origanum vulgare*).

SPANISH OREGANO FLOWERS

*A perennial creeping herb with a woody stem, small dark green leaves, and pink or white flowers borne in clusters.*

### DATAFILE

**AROMATHERAPY/ HOME USE**
None. It should not be used on the skin.

**EXTRACTION**
Essential oil by steam distillation from the dried flowering tops.

**ACTIONS**
See Common oregano, page 111.

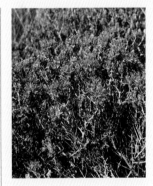

*Thymus capitatus*
*Native to the Middle East and Asia Minor; grows wild in Spain. The oil is produced in Spain, Israel, Lebanon, Syria, and Turkey.*

**SAFETY DATA**
Dermal toxin, skin irritant, mucous membrane irritant

*THYMUS VULGARIS*

# Common thyme

FAMILY: LAMIACEAE (LABIATAE)

## Herbal/Folk Tradition

One of the earliest medicinal plants in Western herbal medicine, its main areas of application are respiratory

problems, digestive complaints, and the prevention and treatment of infection. In the *British Herbal Pharmacopoeia* it is indicated for dyspepsia, chronic gastritis, bronchitis, pertussis, asthma, children's diarrhea, laryngitis, tonsillitis, and enuresis in children.

FRESH THYME

*A perennial evergreen subshrub up to 18in (45cm) high with a woody root and much-branched stem. It has gray-green, aromatic leaves and pale purple or white flowers.*

---

**DATAFILE**

### AROMATHERAPY/ HOME USE

Can irritate mucous membranes, cause dermal irritation and may cause sensitization in some individuals. Use in moderation, in low dilution only. Best avoided during pregnancy.
**Skin Care:** *Abscess, acne, bruises, burns, cuts, dermatitis, eczema, insect bites, lice, gum infections, oily skin, scabies.*
**Circulation, Muscles, and Joints:** *Arthritis, cellulitis, gout, muscular aches and pains, obesity, edema, poor circulation, rheumatism,*
*sprains, sports injuries.*
**Respiratory System:** *Asthma, bronchitis, catarrh, coughs, laryngitis, sinusitis, sore throat, tonsillitis.*
**Digestive System:** *Diarrhea, dyspepsia, flatulence.*
**Genitourinary System:** *Cystitis, urethritis.*
**Immune System:** *Chills, colds, flu, infectious diseases.*
**Nervous System:** *Headaches, insomnia, nervous debility, and stress-related complaints.*

### EXTRACTION
Essential oil by water or steam distillation from the fresh or partially dried leaves and flowering tops. "Red thyme oil" is the crude distillate. "White thyme oil" is produced by further redistillation or rectification.

### ACTIONS
Anthelmintic, antimicrobial, antioxidant, antiputrescent, antirheumatic, antiseptic (intestinal, pulmonary, genitourinary), antispasmodic, antitussive, antitoxic, aperitif,
astringent, aphrodisiac, bactericidal, balsamic, carminative, cicatrizant, diuretic, emmenagogue, nervine, revulsive, rubefacient, parasiticide, stimulant (immune system, circulation), sudorific, tonic, vermifuge.

### COMPATIBILITIES
It blends well with bergamot, lemon, rosemary, melissa, lavender, lavandin, marjoram, Peru balsam, and pine.

**SAFETY DATA**
*Contraindicated in cases of high blood pressure. Red thyme oil, serpolet (from wild thyme), "thymol" and "carvacrol" type oils all contain quite large amounts of toxic phenols (carvacrol and thymol). White thyme is not a "complete" oil and is often adulterated. Lemon thyme and "linalol" types are in general less toxic, nonirritant, with less possibility of sensitization – safe for use on the skin and with children*

*TILIA X VULGARIS*

# Linden
FAMILY: TILIACEAE

## Herbal/Folk Tradition
Linden tea, known as "tilleul", is drunk
a great deal in
continental Europe,
as a general relaxant.
The flowers are also
used for indigestion,
palpitations, nausea,
hysteria, and catarrh
following a cold.
Linden honey is
highly regarded.

FRESH LEAVES

*A tall graceful tree up to 98ft (30m) high with a smooth
bark, spreading branches, and bright green, heart-shaped
leaves. It has yellowy-white flowers borne in clusters, which
have a very powerful scent.*

### DATAFILE

**AROMATHERAPY/
HOME USE**
Digestive System: *Cramps,
indigestion, liver pains.*
Nervous System: *Headaches,
insomnia, migraine, nervous tension,
and stress-related conditions.*

**EXTRACTION**
A concrete and absolute by
solvent extraction from the dried
flowers.

**ACTIONS**
Astringent, antispasmodic, bechic,
carminative, cephalic, diaphoretic,
diuretic, emollient, nervine,
sedative, tonic.

*Tilia x vulgaris
Native to Europe and the
northern hemisphere. Common
in Britain, France, and the
Netherlands.*

**SAFETY DATA**
Most products are adulterated or synthetic.
No safety data available at present

---

*TRACHYSPERMUM COPTICUM*

# Ajowan
FAMILY: APIACEAE (UMBELLIFERAE)

## Herbal/Folk Tradition
The seeds are used in curry
powders and as a household
remedy for intestinal problems.
The tincture, essential oil,
and "thymol" are used in India
for cholera.

AJOWAN SEEDS

*An annual herb with a grayish-brown seed. It has bright
green leaves and an erect habit of growth usually not
exceeding 20in (50cm) in height. It is an umbelliferous
plant, widely cultivated in India for medicinal properties.*

### DATAFILE

**AROMATHERAPY/
HOME USE**
Not recommended.

**EXTRACTION**
Essential oil by steam distillation
from the seed.

**ACTIONS**
Powerful antiseptic and
germicide, carminative.

**SAFETY DATA**
Possible mucous membrane and dermal irritant. Due to high thymol level,
should be avoided in pregnancy. Toxicity levels are unknown

*TSUGA CANADENSIS*

# Hemlock spruce

FAMILY: PINACEAE

## Herbal/Folk Tradition

The bark of the hemlock spruce is current in the *British Herbal Pharmacopoeia* indicated for diarrhea, cystitis, mucous colitis, leucorrhea, uterine prolapse, pharyngitis, stomatitis and gingivitis.

NEWLY FORMED CONES

FRESH HEMLOCK SPRUCE | FRESH LEAVES

*A large evergreen tree up to 164ft (50m) tall, with slender horizontal branches, finely toothed leaves, and smallish brown cones. It yields a natural exudation from its bark.*

DATAFILE

### AROMATHERAPY/HOME USE

Circulation, Muscles, and Joints: *Muscular aches and pains, poor circulation, rheumatism.*
Respiratory System: *Asthma, bronchitis, coughs, respiratory weakness.*
Immune System: *Colds, flu, infections.*
Nervous System: *Anxiety, stress-related conditions.*

### EXTRACTION

Essential oil by steam distillation from the needles and twigs.

### ACTIONS

Antimicrobial, antiseptic, antitussive, astringent, diaphoretic, diuretic, expectorant, nervine, rubefacients, tonic.

### COMPATIBILITIES

It blends well with pine, oakmoss, cedarwood, galbanum, benzoin, lavender, lavandin, and rosemary.

### SAFETY DATA
*Nontoxic, nonirritant, nonsensitizing*

---

*VALERIANA FAURIEI*

# Valerian

FAMILY: VALERIANACEAE

## Herbal/Folk Tradition

This herb, highly esteemed since medieval times, has been used in the West for complaints where there is nervous tension, such as insomnia, and migraine, and as a pain reliever.

ROOT OF VALERIAN

*A perennial herb up to 5ft (1.5m) high with a hollow, erect stem, deeply dissected dark leaves, and many purplish-white flowers. It has short, thick, grayish roots, largely showing above ground, which have a strong odor.*

DATAFILE

### AROMATHERAPY/HOME USE

Nervous System: *Insomnia, nervous indigestion, migraine, restlessness, and tension states.*

### EXTRACTION

Essential oil by steam distillation from the rhizomes. An absolute and concrete by solvent extraction of rhizomes.

### ACTIONS

Anodyne, antidandruff, diuretic, antispasmodic, bactericidal, carminative, depressant of the central nervous system, hypnotic, hypotensive, regulator, sedative, stomachic.

*Valeriana fauriei*

### COMPATIBILITIES

It blends well with patchouli, costus, oakmoss, pine, lavender, cedarwood, mandarin, petitgrain, and rosemary.

### SAFETY DATA
*Nontoxic, nonirritant, possible sensitization. Use in moderation*

*VANILLA PLANIFOLIA*

# Vanilla

FAMILY: ORCHIDACEAE

## Herbal/Folk Tradition

When vanilla is grown in cultivation, the deep trumpet-shaped flowers have to be hand-pollinated – except in Mexico where the native humming birds do most of the work!

DRIED VANILLA BEAN

*A perennial herbaceous climbing vine up to 82ft (25m) high, with green stems and large white flowers that have a deep narrow trumpet. The green capsules or fruits are picked and "cured". The immature vanilla "pod" or "bean" is fermented and dried to turn it into a fragrant brown vanilla bean.*

### DATAFILE

**AROMATHERAPY/ HOME USE**
None.

**EXTRACTION**
A resinoid (often called an oleoresin) by solvent extraction from the "cured" vanilla beans. (An absolute is occasionally produced by further extraction from the resinoid.)

**ACTIONS**
Balsamic.

**COMPATIBILITIES**
It blends well with sandalwood, vetiver, opopanax, benzoin, balsams, and spice oils.

*Vanilla planifolia
Native to Central America and Mexico.*

**SAFETY DATA**
Nontoxic, common sensitizing agent. Widely adulterated

---

*VETIVERIA ZIZANIOIDES*

# Vetiver

FAMILY: POACEAE (GRAMINEAE)

## Herbal/Folk Tradition

The rootlets have been used in the East for their fine fragrance since antiquity. They are used by the locals to protect domestic animals from vermin. In India and Sri Lanka the essence is known as "the oil of tranquillity".

FRESH VETIVER GRASS

DRIED VETIVER GRASS

*A tall, tufted, perennial, scented grass, with a straight stem, long, narrow leaves, and an abundant, complex lacework of underground white rootlets.*

### DATAFILE

**AROMATHERAPY/ HOME USE**
Skin Care: *Acne, cuts, oily skin, wounds.*
Circulation, Muscles, and Joints: *Arthritis, muscular aches and pains, rheumatism, sprains, stiffness.*
Nervous System: *Debility, depression, insomnia, nervous tension – Vetiver is deeply relaxing, and is a valuable oil in massage and baths for anybody suffering from stress.*

**EXTRACTION**
Essential oil by steam distillation from the roots and rootlets – washed, chopped, dried, and soaked. A resinoid is produced by solvent extraction for perfumery work.

**ACTIONS**
Antiseptic, antispasmodic, depurative, rubefacient, sedative (nervous system), stimulant (circulatory, production of red corpuscles), tonic, vermifuge.

**COMPATIBILITIES**
It blends well with sandalwood, rose, violet, jasmine, opopanax, patchouli, oakmoss, lavender, clary sage, mimosa, cassie, and ylang ylang.

**SAFETY DATA**
Nontoxic, nonirritant, nonsensitizing

*VIOLA ODORATA*

# Violet

FAMILY: VIOLACEAE

## Herbal/Folk Tradition

Both the leaf and flowers have a long tradition of use in herbal medicine,

mainly for congestive pulmonary conditions and sensitive skin conditions. The leaf has also been used to treat cystitis and as a mouthwash for infections of the mouth and throat.

FLOWERING SPRIG OF VIOLET

*A small, tender, perennial plant with dark green, heart-shaped leaves, fragrant violet-blue flowers, and an oblique underground rhizome.*

### DATAFILE

**AROMATHERAPY/ HOME USE**

**Skin Care:** *Acne, eczema, refiines the pores, thread veins, wounds.*
**Circulation, Muscles, and Joints:** *Fibrosis, poor circulation, rheumatism.*
**Respiratory System:** *Bronchitis, catarrh, mouth and throat infections.*
**Nervous System:** *Dizziness, headaches, insomnia, nervous exhaustion – the scent was believed to comfort and strengthen the heart.*

**EXTRACTION**
A concrete and absolute from fresh leaves or flowers.

**ACTIONS**
Analgestic (mild), anti-inflammatory, antirheumatic, antiseptic, decongestant (liver), diuretic, expectorant, laxative, soporific, stimulant (circulation).

**COMPATIBILITIES**
It blends well with tuberose, clary sage, boronia, tarragon, cumin, hop, basil, hyacinth, and other florals.

**SAFETY DATA**
*Nontoxic, nonirritant, possible sensitization in some individuals*

---

*ZINGIBER OFFICINALE*

# Ginger

FAMILY: ZINGIBERACEAE

## Herbal/Folk Tradition

Ginger has been used as a spice and as a remedy for thousands of years. In China fresh ginger is used for complaints ranging from to malaria to rheumatism. It is best known as a digestive aid.

GROUND GINGER

SECTION OF ROOT

RHIZOME ROOT

*An erect perennial herb up to 3ft (1m) high with a thick, spreading, pungent tuberous rhizome. Each year it sends up a green reedlike stalk with narrow spear-shaped leaves and white or yellow flowers on a spike direct from the root.*

### DATAFILE

**AROMATHERAPY/ HOME USE**

**Circulation, Muscles, and Joints:** *Arthritis, fatigue, muscular aches and pains, poor circulation, rheumatism, sprains, strains, etc.*
**Respiratory System:** *Catarrh, congestion, coughs, sinusitis, sore throat.*
**Digestive System:** *Diarrhea, colic, cramp, flatulence, indigestion, loss of appetite, nausea, travel sickness.*
**Immune System:** *Chills, colds, flu, fever, infectious disease.*
**Nervous System:** *Debility, nervous exhaustion.*

**EXTRACTION**
Essential oil by steam distillation from unpeeled, dried ground, root.

**ACTIONS**
Analgesic, antioxidant, antiseptic, antispasmodic, antitussive, aperitif, aphrodisiac, bactericidal, carminative, cephalic, diaphoretic, expectorant, febrifuge, laxative, rubefacient, stimulant, stomachic.

**COMPATIBILITIES**
It blends well with sandalwood, vetiver, patchouli, frankincense, rosewood, cedarwood, coriander, rose, lime, orange blossom, orange, and other citrus oils.

**SAFETY DATA**
*Nontoxic, nonirritant (except in high concentration), slightly phototoxic; may cause sensitization in some individuals*

# Glossary

**Abortifacient:** capable of inducing abortion.

**Absolute:** a highly concentrated viscous, semisolid, or solid perfume material, usually obtained by alcohol extraction from the concrete.

**Allergy:** hypersensitivity caused by a foreign substance.

**Alterative:** corrects disordered bodily function.

**Amenorrhea:** absence of menstruation.

**Analgesic:** remedy that deadens pain.

**Anemia:** deficiency in either quality or quantity of red corpuscles in the blood.

**Annual:** refers to a plant that completes its life cycle in one year.

**Anodyne:** stills pain and quiets disturbed feelings.

**Anthelmintic:** a vermifuge, destroying or expelling intestinal worms.

**Antibiotic:** prevents the growth of, or destroys, bacteria.

**Antiemetic:** an agent that reduces the incidence and severity of nausea.

**Antihemorrhagic:** an agent that prevents or combats hemorrhage or bleeding.

**Antihistamine:** treats allergic conditions; counteracts effects of histamine (produces capillary dilation).

**Antimicrobial:** an agent that resists or destroys pathogenic microorganisms.

**Antioxidant:** a substance used to prevent or delay oxidation or deterioration, especially with exposure to air.

**Antiphlogistic:** checks or counteracts inflammation.

**Antipruritic:** relieves sensation of itching or prevents its occurrence.

**Antipyretic:** reduces fever.

**Antisclerotic:** helps prevent the hardening of tissue.

**Antiseborrheic:** helps control the products of sebum, the oily secretion from sweat glands.

**Antitoxic:** an antidote or treatment that counteracts the effects of poison.

**Antitussive:** relieves coughs.

**Aperient:** a mild laxative.

**Aphonia:** loss of voice.

**Apoplexy:** sudden loss of consciousness, a stroke, or sudden, severe hemorrhage.

**Aril:** the husk or membrane covering the seed of a plant.

**Aromatherapy:** the therapeutic use of essential oils.

**Arteriosclerosis:** loss of elasticity in the artery walls due to thickening.

**Astringent:** causes contraction of organic tissues.

**Atony:** lessening or lack of muscle tone.

**Axil:** upper angle between a stem and leaf or bract.

**Bactericidal:** an agent that destroys bacteria.

**Balsam:** a resinous semisolid mass or viscous liquid exuded from a plant. A "true" balsam has a high content of benzoic acid, benzoates, cinnamic acid, or cinnamates.

**Balsamic:** a soothing medicine or application.

**Bechic:** anything that relieves or cures coughs; or referring to cough.

**Biennial:** a plant that completes its life cycle in two years, without flowering in the first year.

**Bilious:** a condition caused by an excessive secretion of bile.

**Calmative:** a sedative.

**Calyx:** the sepals or outer layer of floral leaves.

**Capsule:** a dry fruit, opening when ripe, composed of more than one carpel.

**Cardiac:** pertaining to the heart.

**Carminative:** settles the digestive system, relieves flatulence.

**Chemotype:** the same botanical species occurring in other forms due to different conditions of growth

**Cholagogue:** stimulates the secretion and flow of bile into the duodenum.

**Cholecystokinetic:** agent that stimulates the contraction of the gall bladder.

**Choleretic:** aids excretion of bile by the liver, so there is a greater flow of bile.

**Cholesterol:** a steroid alcohol found in nervous tissue, red blood cells, animal fat, and bile.

**Cicatrizant:** an agent that promotes healing by the formation of scar tissue.

**Cirrhosis:** degeneration in any organ (especially liver), caused by various poisons, bacteria, or other agents, resulting in fibrous tissue overgrowth.

**Colic:** pain due to contraction of the muscle of the abdominal organs.

**Colitis:** inflammation of the colon.

**Concrete:** a concentrate, waxy, solid, or semisolid perfume material made from previously live plant matter, usually using a hydrocarbon type of solvent.

**Corolla:** the petals of a flower.

**Cutaneous:** pertaining to the skin.

**Cystitis:** bladder inflammation, usually characterized by pain on urinating.

**Cytophylactic:** the process of increasing the activity of leucocytes in defense of the body against infection.

**Cytotoxic:** toxic to all cells.

**Decoction:** a herbal preparation, where the plant material is boiled in water and reduced to make a concentration.

**Demulcent:** a substance that protects mucous membranes and allays irritation.

**Depurative:** helps combat impurity in the blood and organs; detoxifying.

**Dermatitis:** inflammation of the skin.

**Diuretic:** aids production of urine.

**Drupe:** a fleshy fruit, with one or more seeds, each surrounded by a stony layer.

**Dysmenorrhea:** painful menstruation.

**Edema:** a painless swelling caused by fluid retention beneath the skin.

**Emetic:** induces vomiting.

**Emmenagogue:** induces or assists menstruation.

**Emollient:** softens and soothes the skin.

**Engorgement:** congestion of a part of the tissues, or fullness (as in the breasts).

**Enteritis:** inflammation of the mucous membrane of the intestine.

**Enzyme:** complex proteins that are produced by the living cells, and catalyze specific biochemical reactions.

**Essential oil:** a volatile and aromatic liquid (sometimes semisolid), which generally constitutes the odorous principles of a plant. It is obtained by a process of expression or distillation from a single botanical form or species.

**Febrifuge:** combats fever.

**Fixative:** a material that slows down the rate of evaporation of the more volatile components in a perfume composition.

**Fixed oil:** vegetable oils obtained from plants that are fatty, dense, and non-volatile, such as olive oil.

**Follicle:** a dry, one-celled, fruit.

**Galactagogue:** increases milk secretion.

**Germicidal:** destroys germs or micro-organisms such as bacteria, etc.

**Gums:** The term "gum" is often applied to "resins." Strictly speaking, gums are natural or synthetic water-soluble materials, such as gum arabic.

**Heartwood:** central part of a tree trunk.

**Hematuria:** blood in the urine.

**Hemorrhoids:** piles, dilated rectal veins.

**Hemostatic:** arrests bleeding.

**Hepatic:** relating to the liver.

**Herpes:** inflammation of the skin or mucous membrane.

**Hormone:** a product of living cells that produces a specific effect on the activity of cells remote from its point of origin.

**Hybrid:** a plant created by fertilization of one species or subspecies by another.

**Hypertension:** raised blood pressure.

**Hypocholesterolemia:** lowering the cholesterol content of the blood.

**Hypoglycemia:** lowered blood sugar levels or concentration.

**Hypotension:** low blood pressure, or a fall in blood pressure.

**Inflorescence:** flowering structure above the last stem leaves.

**Infusion:** a herbal remedy prepared by steeping the plant material in water.

**Lanceolate:** lance-shaped, oval, and pointed at both ends.

**Legume:** a fruit consisting of one carpel, opening on one side, such as a pea.

**Leucocyte:** white blood cells responsible for fighting disease.

**Leucocytosis:** an increase in the number of white blood cells above normal limits.

**Leucorrhea:** white vaginal discharge.

**Ligulet:** a narrow protection from the top of a leaf sheath in grasses.

**Lipolytic:** causing lipolysis, the chemical disintegration or splitting of fats.

**Macerate:** soak until soft.

**Menopause:** the normal cessation of menstruation, a life change for women.

**Menorrhagia:** excessive menstruation.

**Metrorrhagia:** uterine bleeding outside the menstrual cycle.

**Microbe:** a minute living organism – pathogenic bacteria, viruses, etc.

**Mucilage:** a substance containing demulcent gelatinous constituents.

**Mucolytic:** breaking down mucus.

**Narcotic:** a substance that induces sleep; intoxicating or poisonous in large doses.

**Nervine:** strengthening and toning to the nerves and nervous system.

**Nephritis:** inflammation of the kidneys.

**Neuralgia:** a stabbing pain along a nerve pathway.

**Neurasthenia:** nervous exhaustion.

**Oleo gum resin:** a natural exudation from trees and plants that consists mainly of essential oil, gum, and resin.

**Oleoresin:** a natural resinous exudation from plants, or an aromatic liquid preparation, extracted from botanical matter using solvents.

**Ovate:** egg-shaped.

**Palpitation:** undue awareness of the heartbeat, occasioned by anxiety. Rapid heartbeats or abnormal rhythm.

**Pappus:** the calyx in a composite flower having feathery hairs, scales, or bristles.

**Parturient:** aiding childbirth.

**Pathogenic:** causing or producing disease.

**Peptic:** applied to gastric secretions and areas affected by them.

**Perennial:** a plant that lives for more than two years.

**Petiole:** the stalk of a leaf.

**Pharmacology:** medical science of drugs.

**Pharmacopoeia:** an official publication of drugs in common use.

**Phytohormones:** plant substances that mimic the action of human hormones.

**Phytotherapy:** the treatment of disease by plants; herbal medicine.

**Pinnate:** a leaf composed of more than three leaflets arranged in two rows along a common stalk.

**Prophylactic:** preventative of disease or infection.

**Prostatitis:** any inflammatory condition of the prostate gland.

**Pruritis:** itching.

**Psoriasis:** a skin disease characterized by red patches and silver scaling.

**Psychosomatic:** the manifestation of physical symptoms resulting from a mental state.

**Pulmonary:** pertaining to the lungs.

**Pyelitis:** inflammation of the kidney.

**Receptacle:** the upper part of the stem from which the floral parts arise.

**Rectification:** the process of redistillation applied to essential oils to rid them of certain constituents.

**Regulator:** an agent that helps balance and regulate the functions of the body.

**Renal:** pertaining to the kidney.

**Resins:** a natural or prepared product, either solid or semisolid in nature. Natural resins are exudations from trees, such as mastic; prepared resins are oleoresins from which essential oil has been removed.

**Resinoids:** a perfumery material prepared from natural resinous matter, such as balsams, by extraction with a hydrocarbon type of solvent.

**Resolvent:** an agent that disperses swelling, or effects absorption of a new growth.

**Rhizome:** an underground stem lasting more than one season.

**Rosette:** leaves that are closely arranged in a spiral.

**Rubefacient:** a substance that causes redness of the skin, possibly irritation.

**Sciatica:** pain down the back of the legs, in the area supplied by the sciatic nerve.

**Sclerosis:** hardening of tissue due to inflammation.

**Seborrhea:** increased secretion of sebum, usually associated with excessive oil secretion from the sweat glands.

**Sessile:** without a stalk.

**Sialogogue:** an agent that stimulates the secretion of saliva.

**Spike:** an inflorescence in which the sessile flowers are arranged in a raceme.

**Splenic:** relating to the spleen, the largest endocrine gland.

**Styptic:** an astringent agent that stops or reduces external bleeding.

**Sudorific:** an agent that causes sweating.

**Synergy:** agents working together harmoniously.

**Tachycardia:** abnormally increased heartbeat and pulse rate.

**Tannin:** an astringent substance that helps seal the tissue.

**Thrombosis:** formation of a thrombus or blood clot.

**Thrush:** an infection of the mouth or vaginal region caused by a fungus.

**Tincture:** a herbal remedy or perfumery material prepared in an alcohol base.

**Tracheitis:** inflammation of the windpipe.

**Trifoliate:** a plant having three distinct leaflets.

**Tuber:** a swollen part of an underground stem of one year's duration, capable of new growth.

**Umbel:** umbrellalike; a flower where the petioles arise from the stem top

**Vermifuge:** expels intestinal worms.

**Volatile:** unstable, evaporates easily, as in "volatile oil"; *see* Essential oil.

**Vulnerary:** an agent that helps heal wounds and sores by external application.

**Whorl:** a circle of leaves around a node.

# Further Reading

ARCTANDER, S. *Perfume and Flavor Materials of Natural Origin,* published by the author, Elizabeth, New Jersey, 1960.

DE BAIRACLI, LEVY, J. *The Illustrated Herbal Handbook,* Faber & Faber, 1982.

BAERHEIM, S.A. & SCHEFFER, J.J.C. *Essential Oils and Aromatic Plants,* Dr. W. Junk Publications, 1989.

BECKETT, S. *Herbs to Soothe Your Nerves,* Thorsons, 1977.

BERESFORD-COOKE, C. *Massage for Healing and Relaxation,* Arlington, 1986.

BIANCHINI, F. & CORBETTA, F. *Health Plants of the World – Atlas of Medicinal Plants,* Newsweek Books, New York, 1977.

BUCHMAN, D.D. *Feed Your Face,* Duckworth, 1980.

BUCHMAN, D.D. *Herbal Medicine,* Rider, 1984.

CHETWYND, T. *A Dictionary of Symbols,* Paladin, 1982.

CHIEJ, R. *The Macdonald Encyclopedia of Medicinal Plants,* Arnoldo Mondadori, Editore, Milan, 1984.

CONWAY, D. *The Magic of Herbs,* Mayflower, 1973.

COON, N. *The Dictionary of Useful Plants,* Rodale, Emmaus, Pa.,1974.

CULPEPER, N. *Culpeper's Complete Herbal,* W. Foulsham & Co. Ltd, 1952.

DAVIS, P. *Aromatherapy, An A–Z,* C.W. Daniel, 1988.

FAY, I. *Perfumery with Herbs,* Darton, Longman and Todd, 1979.

DOUGLAS, J.S. *Making Your Own Cosmetics,* Pelham Books, 1979.

DOWNING, G. *The Massage Book,* Penguin, 1974.

GRIEVE, M. *A Modern Herbal,* Penguin, 1982.

GRIGGS, B. *The Home Herbal,* Pan, 1983.

GUENTHER, E. *The Essential Oils,* Van Nostrand, New York, 1948.

HALL, R., KLEMME D. & NIENHAUS J. *The H & R Book: Guide to Fragrance Ingredients,* Johnson Publishing, 1985.

HEPPER, C. *Herbal Cosmetics,* Thorsons, 1987.

HERITEATU, J. *Potpourris and other Fragrant Delights,* Penguin, 1975.

HOFFMAN, D. *The New Holistic Herbal,* Element Books, 1990.

HUXLEY, A. *Natural Beauty With Herbs,* Darton, Longman and Todd, 1977.

JESSEE, J.E. *Perfume Album,* Robert E. Krieger, 1974.

LAUTIE, R. & PASSEBECQ, A. *Aromatherapy; the Use of Plant Essences in Healing,* Thorsons, 1982.

LAVABRE, M. *Aromatherapy Workbook,* Healing Arts Press, Vermont, 1990.

LAWERENCE, B.M. *Essential Oils,* Allured Publishing Co., Wheaton, USA, 1978.

LEUNG, A.Y. *Encyclopedia of Common Natural Ingredients,* John Wiley, New York, 1980.

LITTLE, K. *Kitty Little's Book of Herbal Beauty,* Penguin, 1980.

MAURY, M. *Marguerite Maury's Guide to Aromatherapy,* C.W. Daniel, 1989.

MABEY, R. *The Complete New Herbal,* Elm Tree Books, 1988.

METCALFE, J. *Herbs and Aromatherapy,* Webb & Bower, 1989.

MILLS, S.Y. *The A–Z of Modern Herbalism,* Thorsons, 1989.

NAVES, Y.R. & MAZUYER, G. *Natural Perfume Materials,* Reinhold Publishing, New York, 1947.

PAGE, M. *The Observers Book of Herbs,* Frederick Warne, 1980.

PRICE, S. *Practical Aromatherapy,* Thorsons, 1983.

ROSE, F. *The Wild Flower Key,* Frederick Warne, 1981.

RYMAN, D. *The Aromatherapy Handbook,* Century, 1984.

STEAD, C. *The Power of Holistic Aromatherapy,* Javelin Books, 1986.

STOBART, T. *Herbs, Spices and Flavourings,* Penguin, 1979.

LE STRANGE, R. *A History of Herbal Plants,* Angus and Robertson, 1977.

THOMSON, W.A.R. *Healing Plants – A Modern Herbal,* Macmillan, 1978.

TISSERAND, R. *The Essential Oil Safety Data Manual,* The Association of Tisserand Aromatherapists, 1985.

TISSERAND, R. *The Art of Aromatherapy,* C.W. Daniel, 1985.

VALNET, J. *The Practice of Aromatherapy,* C.W. Daniel (English Translation), 1982.

WEISS, R.F. *Herbal Medicine,* Arcanum, 1988.

WHITMONT, E.C. *Psyche and Substance,* North Atlantic Books, 1980.

WILLIAMS, D. *Lecture Notes on Essential Oils,* Eve Taylor Ltd, 1989.

WORWOOD, V.A. *The Fragrant Pharmacy,* Macmillan, 1990.

WREN, R.C. *Potters New Cyclopaedia of Botanical Drugs and Preparations,* C.W. Daniel, 1988.

# References

1. BAERHEIM & SCHEFFER. *Essential Oils and Aromatic Plants.*

2. TISSERAND, R. *The Essential Oil Safety Manual*, p.79.

3. LAVABRE, M. *Aromatherapy Workbook*, p.86.

4. DAVIS, P. *Aromatherapy, An A–Z*, p.135.

5. MONCRIEFF, R.W. *Odours*, 1970.

6. MAURY, M. *Marguerite Maury's Guide to Aromatherapy*, p.104.

7. LEUNG, A.Y. *Encyclopedia of Common Natural Ingredients*, p.155.

8. TISSERAND, as above, p.96.

9. DAVIS, as above, p.236.

10. TISSERAND, as above, p.189.

11. GRIEVE, M. *A Modern Herbal*, p.127.

12. LEUNG, A.Y. *Encyclopedia of Common Natural Ingredients*, p.166.

13. GRIEVE, as above.

14. MAURY, as above, p.104.

15. TISSERAND, as above, p.84.

16. CULPEPER, N. *Culpeper's Complete Herbal*, p.202.

17. TISSERAND, R. *The Art of Aromatherapy*, p.238.

18. ARCTANDER, S. *Perfume and Flavor Materials of Natural Origin*, p.581.

19. CULPEPER, as above, p.211.

20. DAVIS, as above, p.328.

21. SCHOOL OF HERBAL MEDICINE, *Materia Medica, Part II*, p.25.

22. HOFFMANN, D. *The New Holistic Herbal*, p.168.

23. CULPEPER, as above, p.298.

24. *British Herbal Pharmacopoeia 1983*, p.181.

25. ARCTANDER, as above, p.563.

26. LEUNG, as above, p.62.

27. ARCTANDER, as above, p.607.

# Useful Addresses

A wide selection of top-quality essential oils, base oils, aromatherapy books, and other aromatic products is available from Aqua Oleum UK. International mail order professional and export lists are also offered. Safety information, quality control, and up-to-date product data are outlined in *The Essential Oil Catalogue* supplied free with price list.

**Aqua Oleum**
Unit 3, Lower Wharf, Wallbridge,
Stroud, Glos GL5 3JA, UK
Tel (01453) 753555
Fax (01453) 752179

*Aqua Oleum products are also available from:*

## CANADA & USA
**Nature Trading Limited**
Box 263, 1857 West 4th Avenue,
Vancouver, B.C., Canada, V63 1M4

## DENMARK & SWEDEN
**Urtekram A/S**, Klostermarken 20,
DK-9550 Mariager, Denmark

## FINLAND
**Luonnonruokkatukku**
Aduki Ky, Kirvesmelhankatu 10,
00810 Helsinki, Finland

## IRELAND
**Wholefoods Wholesale**
Unit 2D, Kylemore Industrial Estate,
Dublin 10, Republic of Ireland

**Soap Opera Ltd**
Unit 3, Enterprise Centre,
Stafford Street, Nenagh,
Co. Tipperary, Republic of Ireland

## JAPAN
**Marunake K.K.**
1-12-4 Ginza Chuo-ku, Tokyo, Japan

## HONG KONG
7 Old Bailey Street, Central,
Hong Kong

*Information regarding qualified aromatherapists and training programmes can be obtained from:*

## UK
**The International Federation of Aromatherapists**
Stamford House, 2/4 Chiswick High Road, London, W4 1TH, UK
Tel: 020 8742 2605

## USA
**The American Alliance of Aromatherapy**
PO Box 750428, Petaluma,
CA 94975, USA
Tel: (707) 778 6762

## AUSTRALIA
**The International Federation of Aromatherapists**
1/390 Burwood Road, Hawthorne,
Melbourne, Victoria 3122, Australia
Tel: (613) 819 2502
Fax: (613) 819 2399

*Information regarding qualified medical herbalists and training programs can be obtained from:*

## UK
**The School of Herbal Medicine/Phytotherapy**
Bucksteep Manor, Bodle Street Green,
Hailsham, Sussex, BN27 4RJ, UK
Tel: (01323) 833 812/4

**The National Institute of Medical Herbalists**
56 Longbrook Street, Exeter,
Devon, EX4 6AH, UK
Tel: (01392) 426022

## USA
**American Botanical Council and Herb Research Foundation**, PO Box 201660, Austin, Texas 78720, USA

**California School of Herbal Studies**
9309 HWY 116, Forestville, CA 95436, USA

## AUSTRALIA
**National Herbalists Association of Australia**, Suite 305, 3 Smail Street, Broadway, New South Wales 2007, Australia
Tel: (02) 211 6437
Fax: (02) 211 6452

*General information on holistic forms of treatment can be obtained from:*

## UK
**British Holistic Medical Association**
Trust House, Royal Shrewsbury Hospital South, Shrewsbury, Shropshire, SY3 8XF, UK
Tel: (01743) 261155
Fax: (01743) 353637

## USA
**American Holistic Medical Association**
Suite 201, 4101 Lake Boone Trail, Raleigh, North Carolina 27607, USA
Tel: (919) 787 5146
Fax: (919) 787 4916

## CANADA
**Canadian Holistic Medical Association**
700 Bay Street, PO Box 101, Suite 604, Toronto, Ontario , M5G 1Z6, Canada

## AUSTRALIA
**Australian Natural Therapists Association**, PO Box 308, Melrose Park, South Australia 5039
Tel: 8297 9533
Fax: 8297 0003

# Index